HOW TO AVOID A
HYSTERECTOMY

HOW TO AVOID A
HYSTERECTOMY
by Lynn Payer

An Indispensable Guide to
Exploring All Your Options—
Before *You Consent to a Hysterectomy*

Pantheon Books
New York

This book is dedicated to all the women
whose stories are told within it;
it is also dedicated to the surgeons who,
by performing my two myomectomies,
acknowledged that their primary duty
is to their patient and not to the reigning
medical dogmas of the times.

Library of Congress Cataloging-in-Publication Data
Payer, Lynn.
How to avoid a hysterectomy.
Includes index.
1. Hysterectomy—Popular works.   2. Surgery,
Unnecessary.   I. Title.   [DNLM: 1. Hysterectomy—
popular works, WP 468 P344h]
RG391.P39   1987   618.1'453   86-42984

ISBN 0-394-55511-2

TEXT DESIGN BY QUINN HALL

Manufactured in the United States of America
FIRST EDITION

Contents

Preface

Hysterectomy is an operative procedure which, in the United States, varies in incidence according to geographical location. The indications for this procedure are often very liberally interpreted, and in some instances they are not very convincing. There is little confusion when the indication for hysterectomy is associated with pelvic cancer. However, when hysterectomy is to be performed in response to benign disease, there is much greater disparity in opinion. Some of the advice given in such cases might not always appear to be in the patient's best interest.

Consumers are exerting pressure upon the medical profession. Whether they like it or not, doctors must serve the consumer in a more dedicated manner than ever before. Lynn Payer's book, addressed to all women, reinforces that. While some of my colleagues may object to many of the points Payer presents, there is no denying that she has felt herself to be a near-victim of our medical health care system. Her views, while not always those of a gynecologic practitioner, reflect her experience. Payer addresses the need for a more humanistic approach in considering the plight of women who are faced with hysterectomy. And she argues effectively that hysterectomy may well have some detrimental consequences for women's health and way of life.

Have all the options been explored? Is there a more acceptable approach? Has the woman been appropriately counseled and informed? Physicians generally want to do what is correct. In this book Lynn Payer helps all women ask the appropriate questions, learn the facts, and do what is right.

CELSO-RAMÓN GARCÍA, M.D.

Acknowledgments

I would like to thank everyone who helped me in the writing of this book, including all the doctors who consented to be interviewed. Special thanks to Drs. Celso-Ramón García, Wulf Utian, James Daniell, John Slocumb, Herbert Winston, and John Paul Micha, who were particularly encouraging, and to Drs. García, Micha, Sadja Greenwood, and Robert Kiwi for reading and critiquing chapters in various stages. I take full responsibility, of course, for the accuracy of the information.

I would also like to thank the Endometriosis Association of Greater New York, particularly Maria Menna Perper, for their cooperation, and Edith Bjornson for sharing her extensive information with me. The staffs at the New York Library for Medical Consumers and the Armand Hammer Library at Columbia University's College of Physicians and Surgeons, where I did much of my research, were always helpful and friendly.

The staff at Pantheon—especially Sara Bershtel, Jeanne Morton, and David Sternbach—must be thanked for their patience. Particular thanks go to editor Betsy Amster, who encouraged a frank style and stubbornly insisted that rather than simply presenting my information, I try to make it meaningful to my readers. And special thanks to my agent and friend, Eleanor Wood.

Finally, I would like to thank Josephine Markham for suggesting the title for chapter 1, "The Hysterectomy Hype"; and Evelyn Jacobs, Marcelle Arak, and Hedi Molnar. Thanks also go to my father for being so understanding of the finances of freelance journalism, and to my sister Cheryl.

HOW TO AVOID A
HYSTERECTOMY

Chapter 1

The Hysterectomy Hype

"*She is as free to make such a decision [for hysterectomy], in a fully informed manner, as she is in deciding whether to have her breasts augmented or reduced, her tummy tucked, or her eyes lifted.*" Letter from a gynecologist published in the *Journal of the American Medical Association*, March 4, 1983

"*If you have a psychotic fixation and you go to the doctor and you want these two fingers amputated, he will not cut them off. But he will remove your genitals.*" Lily Tomlin, quoted in *Rolling Stone*, October 24, 1974

I used to think of hysterectomy as an operation undergone by middle-aged, or even old, women. Although my mother had had one in her late thirties—younger than I am now—to the eyes of a teenager even thirty-five seems old.

But as I entered my thirties I didn't feel particularly old. Like many of my generation, I had put off marriage and children in order to do other things while waiting for Mr. Right to come along. Since I was constantly being assured by the press that older women and even women with serious gynecologic problems could have children, I didn't worry too much about the delay.

When I was thirty-three, a routine gynecologic checkup disclosed a mass in my abdomen the size of a grapefruit that was later shown to be a fibroid tumor of the uterus. I had thus become a candidate for what many gynecologists in this country would consider a "necessary" hysterectomy. I later found out I wasn't abnormally young: in the mid-1970s, over 10 percent of U.S. women aged thirty to thirty-four were estimated to have had a hysterectomy, as were nearly 30 percent of women aged forty to forty-four.[1] In fact, 60 percent of hysterectomies in the United States are performed on women under forty-four.[2]

Had I gone ahead and had a hysterectomy, it would have been classed as a "necessary" one, although as we shall see later "necessary" is a meaningless term that should be discarded. But many women have hysterectomies for even less reason than I would have had. Herbert Winston, M.D., a clinical professor of obstetrics and gynecology at Albert Einstein College of Medicine in New York and a second-opinion consultant for Blue Cross– Blue Shield in the Greater New York area, says that he has disagreed with the recommendations for hysterectomy in about 90 percent of the patients who have seen him for second opinions within the past three or four years. Most of the disagreement arose, not because he tends to avoid hysterectomy whenever possible, but because, as he puts it, "The patients who had had the recommendation for the hysterectomy either had no pathology whatsoever or had pathology that was so minimal that it was inexplicable to me how anybody could have recommended surgery."

I wasn't living in this country at the time my fibroids were first diagnosed, but in France, where the hysterectomy rate is much lower than it is here.[3] There, hysterectomy is considered "necessary" in young women only for gynecologic cancers and for severe bleeding that cannot be controlled by any other method. The two French surgeons I saw didn't even mention hysterectomy as a treatment option; instead, they told me that I should have a myomectomy, or operation to remove the fibroid tumor, before it got so big that it might necessitate a hysterectomy. Myomectomy is major surgery, but it is surgery in which the uterus is repaired, not removed. I underwent the myomectomy and recovered easily. My French surgeon told me I could have six such operations without even needing a cesarean section if I later became pregnant.

A few years later, back in the United States, my uterus regrew many more fibroids, and I was told that a second myomectomy would be impossible. I was advised to have a hysterectomy, even though I had few symptoms. But because of my French experience I knew better: myomectomy was not impossible, even a second time. I insisted that if I agreed to any operation, it would be a myomectomy. My surgeon eventually agreed against what he considered his better judgment, and I had the operation when I was thirty-nine, recovering just as easily as I had from the first.

Some eight years and two myomectomies after my initial fibroid was discovered, I can honestly say that the worst part of my experience was not any symptoms from the fibroids, nor was it the two myomectomies. It was the pressure for hysterectomy I was put under by U.S. physicians. When I resisted a hysterectomy for the regrown fibroids I was told I was crazy, that I was not behaving in a mature fashion, that I needed help!

I did need help, although not at all the kind the gynecologists in question thought I needed.

First and foremost, I needed information. I found most of the books written by doctors for women no help at all.[4] If they mentioned myomectomy, it was usually to condemn it, or to say it could be performed only in women under thirty-five, or in women with only one or two fibroids. Luckily, I didn't stop there. A medical journalist by profession, I knew how to go about getting information directly from medical journals. I did find an article about myomectomy written by Francis Ingersoll, M.D., now retired from Harvard Medical School, that gave me hope that a few U.S. gynecologists believed the uterus important enough to save.[5]

But the more research I did, the more I realized how little is known about issues important to women looking into hysterectomy and its alternatives. For example, while gynecologists are pretty certain that one of the female hormones, estrogen, causes fibroids to grow, medical science has never determined whether another female hormone, progesterone, causes them to grow or shrink—a factor of some importance since both hormones are used in birth-control pills, in hormone-replacement therapy, and sometimes even in the treatment of fibroids!

Doctors also don't know what hysterectomy does to the female sexual response, whether different types of hysterectomy will have different effects on it, or indeed much about the female sexual response at all.

They don't know what the long-term effects are of hormone-replacement therapy given when the ovaries are removed during a hysterectomy.

They don't know what substances the uterus produces, or what effect removal of the uterus has on the rest of the body.

They don't know whether the extraordinary protection against heart attacks that women experience prior to the age of natural menopause is due to the presence of the uterus or the ovaries; removing either seems to increase the risk of heart attack.

They don't even know much about menstrual bleeding, or why some women bleed very heavily.

To some extent this ignorance can be forgiven; our bodies are remarkably complex organisms and our reproductive organs among the most complex organs of all. In addition, the most direct way doctors can learn about these processes is to experiment directly on women, something we certainly don't want them to do indiscriminately!

The ignorance can be forgiven, but the bland reassurances given to us by many doctors cannot be.

Most books about hysterectomy written by doctors, for example, reassure us that hysterectomy will have no adverse effect on our sex life. In *Understanding Hysterectomy: A Woman's Guide*, F. G. Giustini, M.D., and F. J. Keefer, M.D., write, "Sexual response is an emotional experience that finds its source in a mind and a heart which is prepared for it."[6] If your sexual response is *only* in your mind and heart, this may be true, but if you feel something a bit lower in the body, read the next chapter!

Giustini and Keefer also note that a woman who is "sound

psychologically should have no long-term emotional effects." Such language, of course, immediately brands anyone who *does* have long-term emotional effects as psychologically unsound and therefore not worth listening to. In fact, as we shall see in the next chapter, there is evidence that over half of women under forty who have hysterectomies suffer emotional effects, in some cases quite severe ones.

Such bland reassurances are particularly hard to forgive when one realizes that fewer than 10 percent of hysterectomies are performed for cancer.[7] If a hysterectomy will save your life or cure symptoms that have been making you miserable, you might not care quite so much about sexual and emotional issues. But when the operation is advocated as equivalent to cosmetic surgery, as a way to eliminate menstruation for the benefit of your husband,[8] or even as a justifiable treatment for disease that could be treated by other means, you—and other women as well— deserve better.

In my own case, besides needing information, I needed a gynecologist who would treat me as a whole person, one who would carefully weigh the probable effects of any treatment not only on my uterus but on my life and health as a whole. Unfortunately, few physicians are trained to think this way. Instead, they are taught that by treating disease aggressively they will automatically be helping the patient. They like to talk about "definitive treatment," which, in the case of gynecologic disease, means taking out all the reproductive organs. They often seem to overlook the fact that some of us might prefer to go on living with our reproductive organs and a bit of disease, particularly if that disease is not going to kill us or make our life too unpleasant.

In general, treating the disease will help the patient only if the disease is worse than the cure. But while gynecologists often consider large fibroids—by far the most common reason hysterectomies are performed—a serious "disease," probably because they can be felt so prominently upon examination, they may or may not bother the patient very much. I've talked to some patients whose fibroids were "cured" by hysterectomy, and they preferred the fibroids.

While this tendency to be more interested in treating disease than in helping patients can be found in doctors of many specialties, it may be particularly common in obstetrician-gynecologists. Diana Scully, in her excellent book on gynecologic residency, *Men Who Control Women's Health*, wrote that among doctors, obstetrician-gynecologists are said to have a "cure complex," deriving satisfaction from surgical intervention and being frustrated by less aggressive medical treatment.[9] One resident quoted by Scully revealed something about fibroids as a disease, as well as the way gynecologists view intervention, when he remarked, "The fibroids, and routine things you see in gyn—the patient is not really suffering too much from this. After the hysterectomy you feel you have really corrected it."

Two aspects of medical care in the United States exacerbate this tendency. One aspect is the fragmentation of health care into specialties, with each specialist treating a different part of the person. Gynecologists tend not to see the effects of their hysterectomies, which may end up being treated by internists, urologists, or psychiatrists. The internist may not link a patient's heart attack to her hysterectomy several years before, since it is only well-controlled observations of large numbers of women over a long period of time that establish such links.

Another aspect is the fact that medical practices operate much as businesses, and unfortunately gynecologists and surgeons often try to sell hysterectomies because that is what they have in stock. Many of the alternatives require greater surgical skill, and many gynecologists, if they were to take them seriously, would either have to update their skills or refer patients to other doctors. A good doctor will, of course, do this. But there is a powerful financial incentive not to.

The relationship of money to hysterectomy is not a simple one, however. Fee-for-service medicine, where doctors are paid for each service they perform, has often been cited as a cause of the high U.S. hysterectomy rate. But the spread of health maintenance organizations (HMOs), which do not pay doctors for each service, may not improve matters. Fee-for-service medicine provides an incentive to perform as many services as possible, and if hysterectomy is the only service the doctor knows how to perform, then he or she will have an incentive to perform hysterectomies. HMOs, on the other hand, provide incentives to treat the patient as inexpensively as possible. In some cases hysterectomy is cheaper than alternatives such as myomectomy, which costs about the same but may have to be repeated. HMOs will probably help cut down on the number of hysterectomies performed when absolutely nothing is wrong with the patient, but they may make it even harder to find good alternatives when some form of treatment is necessary.

The gynecologist I eventually found in the United States to perform my second myomectomy shared the disease orientation of his colleagues, but he was a good surgeon and an honorable person. While he protested all the way, he did eventually perform the operation that I felt was the best choice for me despite the fact that it was more work for him.

As a woman who has faced hysterectomy I am not alone; if the operation continues to be performed at the current rate, approximately half the women in this country will eventually undergo one, and perhaps every woman will at some time in her life have a hysterectomy recommended to her.[10] Because I knew that most women have trouble getting the information they need, I decided to write the book I would have liked to have had myself a few years earlier.

Books about hysterectomy tend to fall into two groups: those written by women who have had hysterectomies, and those written by doctors, to which I have already alluded. The books by women are directed at helping women who are either reconciled to a hysterectomy or have already had the surgery. The books written by gynecologists, with few exceptions, are written not to inform women but to reassure them—to talk them into hysterectomies, if you will. Because of this, the authors often seem to feel no need to research the issue much beyond what they learned during their medical training.

This book is different. First, I've written it from the point of view of women who want to avoid hysterectomy if at all possible. Second, I've researched as many alternatives as I could, consulting not just any gynecologists but gynecologists who are experts in their fields. Third, I've tried to separate medical facts from medical opinions.

That last point in particular deserves some explanation. In gathering the "facts," I had to resist the efforts of some gynecologists I interviewed to confuse fact with opinion. That fibroids might recur after myomectomy is a fact; that hysterectomy is therefore preferable to myomectomy is an opinion. That certain conditions of the cervix, if untreated, increase the risk of invasive cancer is a fact; that they should be treated by hysterectomy to remove all risk is an opinion. That ovarian cancer is difficult to treat and will affect about 1 percent of women is a fact; that all healthy ovaries of women over forty undergoing pelvic surgery should be removed is an opinion. I have not excluded all opinions offered by doctors, but I have tried to separate fact from opinion in order to help you make your own decision.

As you read through the book you will see that I don't use the terms "necessary," "indicated," or "unnecessary" when talking about hysterectomy, since these are all opinion words, although you may often hear them spoken in doctors' offices as if they were facts. I don't use them because these terms have very different meanings for physicians and for patients. For a woman, a "necessary hysterectomy" usually means that the operation is imperative to save her life and that there are no other alternatives. For the physician, a "necessary hysterectomy" often means simply that some abnormality can be found. The word "indicated" is often used as a synonym for "necessary." "Indicated" is a better term, because it conveys less urgency, but it too can be used to keep a patient from participating in one of the most important decisions ever made about her body. One Colorado gynecologist, for example, reported a series of hysterectomies in which 80 were "indicated" and 253 were "patient-indicated."[11] He explained that for the "patient-indicated" hysterectomies he had carefully discussed the need for the operation with the woman, whereas for the "indicated" hysterectomies "there really is no need for discussion." But when we look at his "indications" for hysterectomy, we find that 19 were performed for large fibroid tumors, 16 for cervical carcinoma-in-situ (in fact, a precancerous condition and not a true cancer), and 11 for heavy bleeding resulting in anemia. As we will see in the chapters that follow, these were all situations where hysterectomy was an *option*—but not by any means the *only* option.

Despite the tendency of physicians to recommend treatment in the first person plural—"We do this; we don't do that"—there is in fact a tremendous difference in the way individual doctors treat the same disease. This is not because some are right and others are wrong—in many cases, it's simply a difference of opinion. There are clearly treatments that *are* wrong, but usually it's more difficult to decide which of several alternative treatments is right. Two perfectly competent and well-educated physicians may look at exactly the same facts and reach diametrically opposed conclusions, perhaps owing to the way they were educated or to their personal experiences. If they were taught to treat disease, they will be more likely to recommend hysterectomy; if they were taught to treat the whole patient, they will be less likely to—or at least, not be as dogmatic about it. If they recently had a patient who died of ovarian cancer that was detected too late, they will be more likely to recommend that all women undergoing hysterectomy over the age of forty have their ovaries out. But if they recently discovered that hormone-replacement therapy when ovaries are removed isn't always all it's cracked up to be, chances are they'll feel the opposite.

The opinions I have included are generally those of gynecologists considered conservative by their peers. This does not mean that they vote Republican, that they adhere to traditional treatments, or that they believe in taking out more organs "just in case." Rather, it means that they tend to believe in leaving the body alone, and if an operation has to be done, in taking out no more than necessary. Some are conservative on some points and more radical on others: one, for example, told me that while he was willing to perform myomectomies on women too old to have children, he felt that anytime he performed a hysterectomy the ovaries should come out at the same time. Overall, as long as I stuck to conservative gynecologists, I was somewhat surprised and pleased that, at least among them, the trend seems to be moving away from hysterectomy to more conservative treatment.

This trend is apparent even in the treatment of cancers of the uterus and ovaries. While conservative gynecologists who do not normally treat cancer said they considered cancer the one instance where they would unequivocally recommend hysterectomy, I found by speaking with gynecologic cancer specialists that there is a revolution going on in the treatment of these cancers similar to the one that began a few years ago in the treatment of breast cancer. Now, as we'll see in chapters 7 and 8, many women with cancer can keep at least some of their reproductive organs.

Among most doctors, however, even those who are conservative, the psychological and sexual consequences of hysterectomy are still not taken very seriously. If you are young and want to have children, you should have little trouble finding gynecologists willing to look at alternatives to hysterectomy. If you are older, though, conservative gynecologists may favor alternatives to hysterectomy only as long as they are less serious procedures. They can understand preferring minor surgery to major surgery, and they can understand wanting to have children, but they have more trouble understanding that older women can have serious psychological and sexual side effects from hysterectomy, or that they may prefer to keep their ovaries even if they do have a hysterectomy.

I have also interviewed a number of women who have faced hysterectomy and managed, in many cases, to avoid it. I recruited them through friends, friends of friends, gynecologists, the Library for Medical Consumers in New York, and the Endometriosis Association of Greater New York. Not only did these women help me determine which facts they most wanted to know about their conditions, but they provided wonderful role models for all of us in dealing with doctors. Several had to stand up to a doctor to insist that their needs and desires be taken into account, and most of them found it as hard as I did. All of them shared their experiences freely in the hope that they will help you. Some of them requested that their names be changed, but all of their stories are real. (In the chapters that follow, I realize that in referring to women by first names and doctors by full name and title, I reflect the pernicious habit that doctors have of addressing us by our first names while we must call them Dr. So-and-So. My intent, however, is not to maintain a woman's subordination to her gynecologist; it is, rather, to protect the identity of the women I interviewed and to fully identify the gynecologists I am quoting.)

A word about organization: You may not want to read this book from cover to cover, but will probably want to read only those chapters relevant to your particular problems. In that case, you may need to skim several chapters, since many conditions occur together. Whatever your problem, you will certainly want to read chapter 3, which outlines specific strategies for avoiding hysterectomy. That chapter and chapter 2, which discusses the side effects of hysterectomy, both contain information that most doctors are not going to tell you.

In the chapters on specific problems I have started with fibroids and bleeding because they are by far the most common reasons women have hysterectomies. I've then grouped a number of cancerous and precancerous conditions in the following chapters. Pelvic inflammatory disease, endometriosis, and excessive pain are all closely related, so these three chapters are placed together. Uterine prolapse comes last—but not least.

For each condition, I've attempted to determine what I had wanted to know for my fibroid tumors: for a woman who wishes to retain her uterus, what is at stake? I hope that the information I have found will be useful not only to the woman who is highly motivated to avoid hysterectomy, but also to the one who would simply like more information in order to make an informed decision.

I have tried to define difficult terms the first time they appear in the text. If you need to, you can also refer to the glossary on pages 180–83 for help.

Chapter 2

The Side Effects
of Hysterectomy
and Ovarian Removal

"Menstruation is a nuisance to most women, and if this can be abol-
ished without impairing ovarian function it would probably be a bless-
ing to not only the woman but to her husband." Novak's Textbook of
Gynecology, 1975

"The insides of me felt like a bowl of mush." Letter from a woman
describing how she felt after her hysterectomy

"I've been ripped off before. I'm used to it." A woman describing her
hysterectomy

Eleanor, a historian in her mid-forties, found she had gained weight,
needed to urinate frequently, and was generally dragging. One day after
she had given a lecture, she sat in her car for ten minutes before she
could start the ignition. She made an appointment with her internist
about a month before her annual checkup was due. He examined her,
looked away, and told her she needed a hysterectomy. "You're forty-
five," he said, "not planning to have any more children, and your uterus
is the size it would be if you were two-and-a-half months pregnant. You
have a big fibroid." He told her to see the gynecologist at the HMO
immediately.

 The gynecologist also told her she needed a hysterectomy and talked
baby talk to her—"he used an expression for taking a leak, something

like going pee-pee"—something she had never even done with her two children when they were small. When she asked if hysterectomy might precipitate psychological problems he said, "No, no, it's all in the head," gesturing there with his finger. She flew to San Francisco to see a woman gynecologist, who was much nicer, told her her fibroids were "cute," but also recommended hysterectomy. A third gynecologist, back home, said the same thing. All also recommended that she have her ovaries out to reduce the chance that they might someday become cancerous. Since she had known women who had died of ovarian cancer, this made sense to her, although a friend suggested that by the same token doctors might remove the brain to remove the danger of brain cancer.

After the surgery, Eleanor became infected with five different germs and was in the hospital twelve days instead of the five she had anticipated. What was her experience like after she came home from the hospital? "Well, they never tell you about that. I went back to my writing and sometimes nothing came for weeks on end. Sometimes I don't know what to write, but it doesn't go on for that long. I couldn't hold ideas, and nothing seemed terribly important." When she tried to bring this up with her surgeon, he wasn't interested in hearing about it, although at one point he began opening up to her about the problems he was having with his divorce. "The only thing he asked afterwards was did I have any night sweats, flushes, stuff like that that could be controlled by the estrogens. Once I mentioned I had a crick in my left side. He didn't want to hear about that." In fact, she was having night sweats but they bothered her so little she hadn't realized what they were. When she suggested to the staff at his office that they didn't do a very good job preparing patients for the aftermath of hysterectomy, they said, "But we've got a brochure!"

She did get help from her friends, many of whom suddenly told her they had had hysterectomies and "it takes time." The second year following surgery was better, and now, two years later, Eleanor feels fine, although she thinks some women she's met who've had hysterectomies never quite recover. "I think it takes very hard work. I feel sorry for women who don't work and go through it. I don't know what they do the rest of their lives."

Eleanor believes that in her case there was no alternative, but she cautions women against having the operation unless there is a very *good reason. "I can't understand women doing it so they won't have periods any more—let me tell you that!"*

Eleanor's story shows hysterectomy to be the tradeoff that many women have found it to be. While it is now rare to die of a hysterectomy—about one out of every thousand women do, usually women who are sicker when they have the surgery in the first place—complications are common.[1]

One study of hysterectomy in Manitoba found a 4 percent risk of complications requiring a hospital readmission during the two years following hysterectomy.[2] And while the women in the study visited their gynecologists less frequently for gynecologic problems following their hysterectomy, they visited them more frequently for psychological problems, urinary tract infections, and menopausal symptoms.

Some of the complications are due to removal of the uterus alone, an operation that is known as total hysterectomy. During a hysterectomy, the ovaries are also often removed, an operation known as oophorectomy, which leads to even more complications. In the following discussion of side effects, I have tried to separate the complications of hysterectomy alone from the complications of hysterectomy with bilateral (two-sided) oophorectomy. This is important, since physicians may try to reassure you that hysterectomy by itself will cause no problems, or that hormone therapy can perfectly replace the hormones supplied by the ovaries. But as I found, reading the medical reports and talking to women who have had hysterectomies gives a more complex picture. Some women do feel better after their hysterectomies, particularly if they were having serious symptoms beforehand. And some women do well on hormone-replacement therapy. But not everyone does, and you should understand that there are no guarantees—*before* you agree to have your uterus or ovaries removed.

THE SIDE EFFECTS OF HYSTERECTOMY ALONE

Like any surgical procedure, hysterectomy may cause fevers and infections immediately after the operation. These can usually be treated satisfactorily with antibiotics, but they can prolong the hospital stay and are occasionally life-threatening.

A particularly serious and fairly common complication of hysterectomy is injury to the bladder or one of the ureters, the tubes leading from the kidneys to the bladder. In a *total* hysterectomy—the usual operation in the United States—the cervix is removed, which means the surgeon has to cut very close to your bladder and ureters. (*Subtotal* hysterectomy, an operation sometimes performed in Europe, does not remove the cervix, and is less likely to cause urinary complications.)[3] If the bladder or ureter is actually cut, further surgery may be necessary. One friend of mine needed six major operations in the month after her hysterectomy to correct a severed ureter; another woman won a malpractice suit because it took three corrective operations to stop a leak of urine that required her to use about a hundred Kotex pads per week.[4]

Luckily, such major problems are relatively rare. But more subtle injury to the urinary tract appears to be fairly common, which is particularly ironic, since physicians often cite possible injury to the urinary tract by fibroids to justify performing hysterectomies. In one group of thirty-five Danish women, some found their bladder control had improved following their hysterectomy, but almost an equal number found it had deteriorated.[5] And when x-rays from before and after surgery were compared, they showed that bladder problems had actually gotten worse for the group as a whole; the authors of the paper speculate that as time passes these women may have even more problems controlling urination.

You may also develop crampy, bloated feelings. "Gastrointestinal symptoms are notorious following hysterectomy," says Celso-Ramón García, M.D., head of the department of gynecology at the University of Pennsylvania Medical Center. In general,

he says, the more extensive the operation, the greater the likeli-
hood of such problems—perhaps because the bowel has to fill
more space in the abdomen, or because the scar tissue from the
operation is restricting the normal movements of the bowel.

*Cherri, a retailer in New Mexico, had a hysterectomy eight years
ago when she was thirty for endometriosis, a condition where the lining
of the uterus migrates onto the surface of other organs and bleeds along
with the uterus each month, causing extremely painful cramping and
other symptoms. While the hysterectomy and removal of one ovary cured
her endometriosis, her bowel was clipped during the operation, which
she believes led to her developing diverticulitis (inflammation of the lower
bowel). She also had a large amount of scar tissue that irritated her
abdomen. "This would irritate the diverticulitis, which in turn would
irritate my stomach, and I couldn't do anything. I'd go for weeks without
having a bowel movement. And if I had one, I had bleeding." Cherri's
pain was eventually partially controlled with medication and trigger-
point injections. (See chapter 10.)*

Most doctors doubt that hysterectomy causes diverticulitis,
but the operation may make certain complications of the disease
more likely. One such complication occurs when the bladder and
bowel stick together, allowing a hole or fistula to form between
the two. Fistulas due to diverticulitis are ordinarily more common
in men because in women the uterus stands between the bowel
and bladder. But once you have had a hysterectomy, you lose
this protection and run the risk of developing this complication
as often as men do.[6] Fortunately, the complication is rare in either
sex.

Adhesions, or scar tissue, can lead to bowel symptoms; they
can also lead to pain. A significant proportion of women who
develop chronic pelvic pain do so following hysterectomy.[7]

HYSTERECTOMY AND THE HEART

Nonsmoking women under the age of fifty hardly ever have heart attacks. Although they do begin to have them around fifty, they still have a much lower rate than men of the same age. If a woman under fifty does have a heart attack, it is usually because she is a heavy cigarette smoker or because she has stopped menstruating, either naturally or by having had a hysterectomy.

Physicians still don't know whether it is the menstruating uterus or the ovaries that protect women from heart attacks, although most believe that it is the hormones produced by the ovaries. But at least some evidence indicates that hysterectomy alone, even if the ovaries are retained, will lead to a higher rate of heart attack.

An early study, for example, compared women who had had their uterus and ovaries removed with those who had had only a hysterectomy.[8] They found no difference in the amount of heart disease in the two groups. Most people interpreted this to mean that the ovaries did not protect against heart disease, but the scientists who looked most closely noticed something else: both groups had a higher rate of heart attack than would be expected for women of the same age.

This question was examined more closely in Framingham, Massachusetts, where a sample of the population was carefully followed over a long period of time to see what factors might predict heart disease. Very precise records were kept on the women of Framingham, so it was known exactly who had had only a hysterectomy and who had had her ovaries removed too. When these data were analyzed, they showed that women who had had a hysterectomy, regardless of whether their ovaries were retained or not, tripled their risk of heart attack in the years between their surgery and the time of expected menopause.

These results were published in the late 1970s.[9] Recently I called William Kannel, M.D., then director of the study, to find out whether the results were still valid. Dr. Kannel, now a professor of medicine at Boston University School of Medicine, confirmed that the Framingham results continued to show a protective effect of the uterus on heart disease. He explained that there are two ways the presence of the menstruating uterus might protect the heart. "One is that [the uterus] has been found to produce the substance prostacyclin, which keeps the blood platelets from getting sticky and also dilates blood vessels. The other is that menstruating women have lower hemoglobin and hematocrits (red blood cell counts) than other women, and that people with low hematocrits and hemoglobin tend to have less coronary artery disease and lower blood pressure."

The problem with the Framingham data is that the numbers are small. An alternative explanation for these results is that hysterectomy in some cases can damage the ovaries so that they cease to function. Another study of a large number of nurses reached by questionnaire showed that while ovarian removal before the age of thirty-five increased the risk of heart attack dramatically if hormone-replacement therapy was not used, hysterectomy alone increased the risk only slightly.[10]

So, at present, nobody really knows for sure whether the menstruating uterus protects against heart attacks. But if it is eventually found to provide only a small degree of protection, leaving the uterus in could save more lives from heart attack than removing it saves from uterine cancer. While heart attack is less common in women than men, it is still the number one killer of women over forty. By contrast, only about 4 percent of female deaths in the United States are due to all cancers of the uterus and ovaries combined.

The finding that the uterus secretes substances such as prostacyclin disputes the notion, long cherished by the medical profession, that it is only an organ to hold babies. Scientists are now beginning to study some of the effects of substances secreted by the uterus on the rest of the body, particularly the brain and the other endocrine organs, and are finding that these effects maybe considerable, at least in animals. Dr. János Biró, for example, of the Karolinska Hospital in Stockholm, Sweden, found that removal of the uterus in animals caused some of the endocrine organs to grow and others to shrink, and that giving the animals an extract made of uterine tissue reversed these effects.[11] Harry Ahdieh, Ph.D., a neuroendocrinologist at the Institute for Animal Behavior in Newark, New Jersey, says it's already clear that an animal's uterus not only synthesizes a number of chemicals but also metabolizes the steroid hormones. If the uterus is removed, the blood level of these steroids will rise, he says. "The uterus is not a bag. It's an extremely active organ."

So far, no one quite knows whether the human uterus plays such an active role in the endocrine system as a whole. Some women, however, do report a wide variety of menopausal symptoms when they have had a hysterectomy even if they have kept their ovaries, and this might explain why.

HYSTERECTOMY AND CHILDBEARING

The inability to bear children is the one side effect that every woman who has a hysterectomy will suffer. For some women this will be viewed as a relief, but for others it can be a real tragedy. The National Center for Health Statistics in Washington, D.C., found that about three-quarters of a million married women in America in 1976 who had had hysterectomies still wanted children.[12]

Adoption is sometimes an option, but if you are contemplating a hysterectomy and still want children, you should know that there are from 60 to 100 couples waiting for each available healthy infant.[13]

While gynecologists in the past were accused of wanting to reduce women to the role of incubators, today you may find them insensitive to your desire for children. This is particularly true if you already have children, are single, or are somewhat older than the gynecologist feels is optimal for childbearing.

When my U.S gynecologist was trying to talk me into a hysterectomy for my regrowth of fibroids, one of his arguments was that I didn't have a partner. He was a specialist in the treatment of infertility, and I had chosen him, not because I was trying to get pregnant, but because I felt he would have more expertise in judging when another myomectomy was warranted. The problem with going to an infertility specialist if you are only trying to preserve your fertility, though, is that some may treat you as a second-class citizen. A married women of my age would probably have had no trouble getting a second myomectomy, and when one reads of the number of procedures that some infertility patients undergo it truly boggles the mind. I still feel that my gynecologist had trouble accepting that my health and happiness alone were important enough to justify a second myomectomy.

Even women who don't particularly want children may find they don't like the finality that hysterectomy brings.

One Sunday afternoon while I was working on this book, friends persuaded me to drop it for a few hours to come to a talk in the neighborhood, which turned out to be given by Lynda, a photographer, who we all agreed was a lovely and interesting woman.

I met Lynda on the street several days later, introduced myself, and explained a bit about my work. When I told her I was doing a book on alternatives to hysterectomy, she said, "Well, it's too late for me."

Lynda, it turns out, was just coming out of an intense depression following her hysterectomy at age thirty-seven. I would not have predicted in advance that Lynda would have had such an intense reaction, because she claimed she didn't want children and she had suffered severe symptoms before the hysterectomy—nearly constant bleeding since the age of twenty, hemorrhaging, dizziness, and weakness. When she had had previous gynecologic surgery at twenty-three for a hemorrhaging ovarian cyst, she had pleaded with her doctors to "take everything out," to stop the pain and bleeding, which they refused to do. Her present gynecologist had not pressured her into hysterectomy and she had nothing but praise for him and the hospital where it was performed. She had decided it was time for the hysterectomy when she hemorrhaged during a concert at Carnegie Hall.

But when she woke up from the surgery, Lynda explained, she felt, "What have I done to myself? I felt twenty-five going into the operation and seventy-five coming out of it." For two months following the surgery, she thought about killing herself. She felt better for a while, then

crashed again. Now, after undergoing intensive therapy that her thera-
pist feels might have been more effective if she'd started it before making
the decision for hysterectomy, she is putting her life together again,
spending a year on a fellowship at a major university. She has also
started meeting men again. But while the men she went with when she
was younger never particularly wanted children, the men of her own age
she's meeting now do. "When I was younger," she says, "neither I nor
the men I met were ready to think about having children, but by my mid-
thirties it became an issue, both for me and the men I met who were
single." While Lynda still doesn't know if she would have had children
had she not had the hysterectomy, it is the first time in her life that she
feels one of her options has been irrevocably taken away.

Lynda's reaction may seem extreme, but it is not at all uncommon. Despite the assurances of most doctor-written books
that a well-adjusted woman should have no problems, several
studies that have attempted to follow up women after their hysterectomies have shown a very high rate of depression and other
psychiatric illness.

For example, Dr. D. H. Richards, an English general practitioner, found that when he compared the women in his practice
who had had hysterectomies with those who had had other operations, 70 percent of the hysterectomy patients, compared to
30 percent of women who had undergone other operations, suffered depression within three years of their operation.[14] Nearly
70 percent also suffered hot flashes whether or not their ovaries
had been removed, as well as urinary symptoms and extreme
tiredness. About half had headaches, dizziness, or insomnia.
While women who had had other operations recovered in three
months, hysterectomy patients on the average took nearly a year.
Depression was most common in women who had their hysterectomies before the age of forty.

Many gynecologists are unaware that their patients have
been having such problems, partly because women tend not to
want to tell them. For example, in one study of women who had
been treated for cancer of the cervix, 78 percent of the women
indicated that they presented themselves to their male physicians

as being self-sufficient, brave, courageous, and quite able to manage their own feelings.[15] But almost without exception, they fell apart emotionally for brief periods and sought support and comfort from a female relative or friend and from the female interviewers.

Nancy Kaltreider, M.D., a psychiatrist, and her co-workers at the Langley Porter Institute at the University of California in San Francisco researched women under forty who had undergone hysterectomy for reasons other than cancer.[16] About half of them had their hysterectomy for mild dysplasia of the cervix, a condition which can almost always be treated by less radical means (see chapter 7).

About 60 percent of these women were suffering a degree of what Dr. Kaltreider calls the stress response syndrome, which includes nightmares, altered self-image, depression, and other symptoms. While 43 percent of the women were judged to have mild symptoms, 18 percent had severe ones. One thirty-three-year-old woman, for example, who had had a hysterectomy for abnormal bleeding, wanted nothing more to do with her children, even though before her operation they had been her greatest pleasure. Others who had not had children described feelings of incredible sadness when they saw the children of others.

A similar study in Israel showed that nearly half of patients showed symptoms such as depression, anxiety, loss of libido, or various physical symptoms following hysterectomy.[17] Only 16.2 percent showed such symptoms following removal of their gallbladder. The Israeli authors concluded that such a high rate of complications "surely calls for some soul-searching. No surgeon today would tolerate a similar incidence of postoperative wound infection, although this latter condition is usually less disabling and more responsive to therapy."

HYSTERECTOMY AND SEX

In the study described above, a few of the patients experienced a total loss of ability to experience orgasm, with no signs of improvement after half a year or more.

Because depressive reactions are so common, many physicians and others think that the loss of sexual feeling many women complain of following hysterectomy must be due to depression. As Susanne Morgan, author of *Coping with a Hysterectomy*, says, "Depression doesn't make sex good."

But there are also plenty of physical reasons why sex may be less satisfying after hysterectomy, and some women who've had hysterectomies suggested to me that it's actually the less satisfying sex that makes the woman depressed.

In some cases, particularly in the operation known as radical hysterectomy done for cervical cancer, the vagina may be shortened, making intercourse painful.[18] If the hysterectomy is done for the repair of a dropped (prolapsed) uterus, the vagina may have been tightened to the point that intercourse is impossible, apparently a fairly common mistake of inexperienced surgeons.[19] Scar tissue in the vagina left from removal of the cervix may also make intercourse painful.[20]

But even if a hysterectomy is correctly done by a competent surgeon, it still deprives a woman of her uterus. While for many women the primary sexual response seems to be centered in the clitoris, other women report other types of sensations that may be dependent on the presence of the uterus. During sex, the uterus increases in size, moves around, and gyrates on its axis. During orgasm, it contracts at exactly the same intervals as a man's penis does during his orgasm, making uterine contraction the closest equivalent to male orgasm.

"It's nonsense to say that there will be no change in sex following hysterectomy," says Susanne Morgan. "The uterus is a very strong muscle—as any of you who've had menstrual cramps know."

In addition to removing the uterus, the surgeon must cut

blood vessels and nerves during a hysterectomy, and these too may play a role in sexual sensation. As Vicki Georges Hufnagel, M.D., a gynecologist in private practice in Los Angeles, said on a recent Phil Donahue show, "What we do is cut major vessels and arteries that flow to the hormone centers in the body. We really alter the body." [21] Wulf Utian, M.D., director of obstetrics and gynecology at Mt. Sinai Medical Center in Cleveland, Ohio, suggests that this might explain why studies have shown that subtotal hysterectomy, in which the cervix is not removed, causes less interference with sex. [22] "More nerves are cut in a total hysterectomy," he said. While in a total hysterectomy the uterosacral nerves must be cut, in a subtotal they are not. "We don't know mechanically what we're doing to sexuality when we perform a hysterectomy," he added.

Carol Nadelson, M.D., a professor of psychiatry at Tufts University Medical Center in Boston, believes that vaginal hysterectomy, where the uterus is removed through the vagina, may produce more sexual problems than abdominal hysterectomy. [23] "What you hear from clinicians and patients suggests that vaginal hysterectomy does have an adverse effect on sexuality," she said. "I hear it from patients as a psychiatrist and from other psychiatrists. Physiologically and anatomically it makes some sense—the interruption of nerves is different in the two operations."

Dr. Nadelson believes the sexual loss is unrelated to depression. "If it were depression, you wouldn't get a difference with the two operations." She cautions that so far this is only an impression, and as a scientist she hates to go with impressions. To determine whether vaginal and abdominal hysterectomy affect sexuality differently, she said, one would have to study women both before and after their hysterectomies.

So, given what hysterectomy entails, it is quite possible that your sexuality will be affected. In fact, when women are asked about their sex life following hysterectomy, anywhere from 5 to 65 percent say it has gotten worse, with many studies showing about one-third. [24] Many also say their sex life has improved, either because they are no longer afraid of getting pregnant or because the symptoms for which they had the hysterectomy in the first place, such as pain or bleeding, have been alleviated.

Given the evidence, how can physicians deny that hysterectomy will affect sex?

One reason is that male gynecologists seem to look at sex from their own point of view: after hysterectomy women still have a vagina. But one woman who discovered that sex was more than a psychological problem wrote a couple of months after her hysterectomy, "Somehow the experts [have] managed to equate the ability to have sex with enjoying it."

Another reason is that recent sexological dogma has pointed to the clitoris as the only organ in women capable of true sexual response. Since the clitoris is not removed during a hysterectomy, the argument goes, there should be no sexual loss. In fact, sexual researchers now believe that women's sexual response is more complex. Some women experience pleasure when an area within the vagina known as the G spot is stimulated.[25] Some find the rhythmic contractions of the uterus during orgasm pleasurable.[26] Some enjoy the feel of the uterus pressing against the peritoneum, an extremely sensitive tissue that lines the abdominal cavity.[27]

Still another reason for the relative insensitivity of doctors to sexual loss is that few doctors even ask about sexuality following hysterectomy. If they do, women often minimize their problems, just as they do when they're depressed.

Maureen, an assistant vice-president at a major New York bank, had a radical hysterectomy for cervical cancer at the age of thirty-eight. While she was single and would have liked to have children, she was well reconciled to the operation after thoroughly researching the issue as soon as she got her diagnosis. "My feeling was that I was thirty-eight years old, not married, and not likely to be producing children. I examined philosophically the idea of having a child by myself and decided I didn't want to do that. The two choices were to risk having the cancer spread and cause real problems and perhaps dying, and giving up my rather limited opportunities for having children, and it seemed to me there was no decision."

But the radical hysterectomy, which is a more extensive procedure than total hysterectomy, also shortens the vagina, and Maureen found afterward that sex was sometimes painful. When her gynecologist asked about her sex life, however, she assured him it was fine. Luckily for Maureen, the problem eventually resolved itself with time as her vagina stretched.

The desire of physicians to help people and not hurt them, although understandable enough, undoubtedly leads to a good bit of denial on their part. If a woman claims she has been hurt, her doctor may prefer to believe there is something wrong with her rather than with the procedure he performed. Since there is no easy way to restore sexual loss, by saying it is psychological in origin a physician can deny its reality as a problem he is responsible for dealing with. "If physicians don't want to [or cannot] deal with the problem, they tell you to see a psychiatrist," said Dr. Utian. Unfortunately, there is no evidence that women who lose libido and sexual responsiveness after hysterectomy can regain it following psychotherapy, although therapy may help a woman cope with her loss.

Ideally, it wouldn't make any difference if sexual loss following hysterectomy were due to physical or to psychological factors because it would be taken seriously in either case. "For whatever reason, if women tend to become depressed and have psychosexual dysfunction we need to know about it and be concerned about it so that we can take steps to avoid it," Francis Hutchins, Jr., M.D., an associate clinical professor of obstetrics and gynecology at Hahnemann Medical College in Philadelphia, told a section of the 1986 meeting of the American College of Obstetricians and Gynecologists.

But in reality, to say that the loss of sexual feeling is psychological makes it all too easy for women considering a hysterectomy to think that they won't suffer this side effect because they're well balanced emotionally. "Before surgery I believed women who had sex problems did have psychological problems," admitted one woman who realized two months after her own hysterectomy that her sexual loss was not just in her head.

CAN SEXUAL LOSS BE PREDICTED
BEFORE HYSTERECTOMY?

If you're considering having a hysterectomy, one of your main questions is likely to be whether the operation will adversely affect your sexual life.

The outcome is difficult to predict with certainty, according to researcher Edith Bjornson. Common sense, however, suggests that if your sexual response comes mainly from stimulation of the clitoris, you are less likely to have problems following hysterectomy. If, however, you find intercourse itself more pleasurable, with pleasant sensations coming from the uterus or even deeper in the abdomen, you may find that such sensations will be diminished or lost after the operation. A few gynecologists are now coming around to the idea that women should be warned before a hysterectomy that sex may be different so that they may weigh this factor along with others in reaching a decision.

Anthony Labrum, M.D., a professor of psychiatry and of obstetrics and gynecology at the University of Rochester Medical School in Rochester, New York, is an example. "If the woman herself is very conscious of uterine contractions during orgasm, if she's used to getting stimulation from the anterior wall of the vagina and feeling orgasm significantly in the uterus and perhaps not very much from clitoral stimulation, it may mean she and her partner need to reorganize their lovemaking after the hysterectomy if they decide to go ahead with it," he said.

Dr. Labrum said he never makes the decision for hysterectomy himself, but allows the woman and her husband to make it themselves. If a woman is having a significant amount of pain during intercourse, the pleasure may be totally blotted out by the pain and the couple may decide that the advantages of hysterectomy outweigh the possible deleterious effects. "It's a profit-and-loss situation," he said.

Women I spoke to agreed. "I didn't feel that great about having a hysterectomy, but I didn't feel that great about dying either," said one who had a hysterectomy for severe and uncontrollable bleeding at the age of twenty. Another woman, who had a hysterectomy for the endometriosis she had suffered from for years, told a recent session of the Endometriosis Association, "Sex is much more meaningful to me now because I'm not sick all the time."

Janet, forty-seven, an artist, had been bleeding so heavily she became weak and dizzy, and eventually ended up in the hospital for a D & C (dilatation and curettage, or scraping of the inside of the uterus) and three units of blood. Shortly after our first conversation, she decided on a vaginal hysterectomy. By that time I had heard several reports from women of the loss of sexual feeling and had read several papers on it too. Janet seemed so pleased with her doctor and her decision that I hesitated to pass on this information, but I felt I must, since the women who had suffered sexual loss resented the fact that they had not been told before their hysterectomies. Janet's response: "If a lessening of sexual feeling is the worst thing that can happen, I'd just as soon go ahead with the operation. Right now all I need is a bit of tenderness!" Janet had the operation, and in fact noticed no sexual difficulties afterward.

WHAT HAPPENS IF THE OVARIES ARE ALSO REMOVED?

While younger women are often allowed to keep their ovaries when hysterectomy is performed, some 50 percent of women in the United States who have their hysterectomies over the age of forty will have both ovaries removed even if they are healthy.[28] Doctors justify this removal of healthy organs in several ways. One is that one in every seventy women will eventually develop ovarian cancer, a cancer that is difficult to detect and to cure.[29] Most older women who develop ovarian cancer will die of it. (As we shall see in a later chapter, young women have a greater chance of having borderline ovarian cancers, which have a much better prognosis and which can sometimes be treated by removing only one ovary.)

Another justification is that further surgery may be necessary for conditions such as ovarian cysts if the ovaries are not removed.

Still a third justification is that in the menopausal woman the ovaries have outlived their usefulness since they no longer produce hormones. In the woman who hasn't reached menopause, doctors often maintain that hormone-replacement therapy can completely compensate for any hormone deficits.

For all these reasons, some doctors and hospitals make it a policy that all women over forty undergoing abdominal surgery have their ovaries removed. But the decision is yours: whatever the policy of the hospital, they cannot force you to consent to removal of your ovaries if you state your objections clearly to your doctor and in writing on the consent form.

To help you decide whether *you* prefer to have your ovaries removed, let's look at what the ovaries normally do and consider whether hormones can really replace these functions.

Ovaries produce the eggs that fuse with sperm to make a baby. But they also produce a number of hormones that not only help carry the baby to term but also affect other parts of the body whether you're pregnant or not.

The three main types of hormones are estrogens, progesterone, and testosterone. Estrogens are considered the quintessentially female hormones. They are secreted throughout most of the menstrual cycle and cause growth in the lining of the uterus and in the breast tissue; they also affect the brain, the bones, the skin, and the mucous membranes.[30] Progesterone is secreted during the second half of the menstrual cycle and in higher levels during pregnancy. It opposes to some extent the actions of the estrogens, and it keeps in check the proliferation of tissues in the uterus caused by estrogen. This is why progesterone is thought to cut the risk of such estrogen-related cancers as cancer of the endometrium (the lining of the uterus). It also works with estrogen to maintain adequate amounts of calcium in the bones.

In addition, the ovaries excrete small amounts of testosterone and other androgens. These hormones are found in greater amounts in men and are resoponsible for many of the characteristically male traits; in women they help maintain an interest in sex as well as energy and well-being.

While the secretion of estrogens and progesterone declines sharply at natural menopause, the ovaries continue to secrete small amounts of estrogens as well as testosterone well into the years following menopause.[31]

When the ovaries are removed surgically, most hormone production stops abruptly. The level of estrogen and progesterone drops immediately.[32] This drop in turn causes dramatic rises in two other hormones produced by the brain. One, luteinizing hormone (LH), doubles or triples; another, follicle-stimulating hormone (FSH), can increase to fourteen times its normal level. Nobody really understands the consequences of such rises.

If no hormone-replacement therapy is taken, you will undergo all the symptoms of menopause, only more abruptly. Susanne Morgan calls this "menostop" because it is so sudden. And Sonja McKinlay, Ph.D., of the Cambridge Research Center in Cambridge, Massachusetts, found that most of the symptoms associated with menopause are actually those of women who undergo artificial menopause: in her study, women whose ovaries stopped on their own had surprisingly few symptoms.[33]

Once the ovaries are removed, hot flashes (sometimes referred to as hot flushes) and night sweats are likely to occur. The lack of estrogen will cause increasing dryness of the vulva and vagina, which may make intercourse painful or difficult and may lead to itchiness. The skin in the vagina and elsewhere will become thinner.

The lack of estrogen and progesterone may also affect the brain, where estrogens exert a stimulating effect and progesterone a calming one.[34]

Just how common are such side effects in women who don't take hormone replacement? One English study found that of 100 women studied one to thirty-one years after surgery, only 4 of whom were taking estrogen, 62 percent suffered from depression, 48 percent from insomnia, 46 percent from loss of libido, and 38 percent from painful intercourse.[35] Another study showed that women whose uterus and ovaries were removed had more such symptoms than those whose gallbladder was removed, suggesting that the symptoms were directly related to the removal of the ovaries and not simply to the fact of having had an operation.[36]

If your ovaries are removed significantly before the age you would normally undergo menopause and you don't take hormone therapy, you should know that you will be at increased risk for certain types of arthritis, as well as for osteoporosis, the thinning of bones that occurs normally with aging.[37]

You may also be at increased risk for heart attack. As I noted before, it's unclear whether it's the uterus or the ovaries that prevent heart attacks in young women, but one study of a large number of nurses showed that women who had their ovaries removed before the age of thirty-five and didn't take estrogen had seven times the rate of heart attack as women whose ovaries were not removed.[38] The women also had a higher death rate from all causes than other women in their age group. (This statistic should be interpreted cautiously, however, since those women may have been sicker to begin with.)

It should be mentioned that the health effects of ovarian removal are not all negative. Besides preventing ovarian cancer, removing the ovaries at a young age confers some protection— as long as you don't take estrogen-replacement therapy—against breast cancer, which is much more common than cancers of the uterus and ovary combined. Such a consideration might be important if there has been a lot of breast cancer in your family. Susan Love, M.D., director of the breast clinic at Beth Israel Hospital in Boston, explains that the longer the breast is exposed to the hormonal stimulation of estrogen, the greater the risk of breast cancer. Since removal of the ovaries stops such hormonal stimulation, "the younger you have it done, the less chance you're going to have breast cancer," she said. But if your doctor recommends having your ovaries removed for this reason, consider the rest of what Dr. Love says. Without them, or hormonal replacement, you have a much greater chance that "your bones are going to fall apart, you'll have a heart attack and a stroke and everything else. It's not something we ever tell people to do.

And by and large, people who have their ovaries out at a young age are put on replacement hormones and that nullifies any protective effect ovarian removal is going to have on the breast anyway." Recent evidence indicates, in fact, that such women have a somewhat higher incidence of breast cancer than women who keep their ovaries.[39]

DOES HORMONE-REPLACEMENT THERAPY HELP?

When you go through menopause naturally, you can decide at your leisure whether or not you want to try hormone-replacement therapy, and if you find you don't like it for any reason, you can always quit without feeling that you are any worse off. But if you agree to having your ovaries removed surgically, you are in a bind: if you don't take hormone replacement, you risk a number of rather serious medical problems. So it pays to examine closely the question whether hormone replacement is really as good as the hormones naturally produced by your ovaries before you agree to have your ovaries removed.

Estrogen Alone. Estrogen-replacement therapy may nullify the protective effect that ovarian removal has on breast cancer, but it will help ameliorate some of the effects of losing your ovaries. In fact, even those physicians who remain cautious about its use across the board nevertheless prescribe it for women who have had their ovaries out, partly because their symptoms are so much more severe and partly because they don't run the risk of getting uterine cancer, one of the main side effects of estrogen-replacement therapy.

Even short-term use of estrogen will help with menopausal symptoms such as hot flashes and dry vagina.

For the much touted effects of preventing osteoporosis and (possibly) heart attacks, however, short-term use will be inadequate. To decrease the risk of osteoporosis, you should take estrogens at least five or ten years past the age when menopause would have occurred, usually around the age of fifty. Estrogen *may* decrease the rate of heart attacks both in women whose ovaries have been removed and in women who undergo menopause naturally. However, while some studies have shown this protective effect, others have shown that estrogen may *increase* the risk of heart attack, so the question remains open. Taking estrogen does seem to bring the elevated mortality rate of the young woman without ovaries back down to normal.

But while estrogen may have positive health benefits and may make you feel better, it will not necessarily help if your sex life has suffered following hysterectomy. If orgasm is less intense without your uterus, hormone replacement won't help. And at least three studies have shown that estrogen replacement will not restore libido lost following hysterectomy.[40]

Because of the evidence that estrogen therapy may actually increase the risk of breast cancer, even women who have had their uterus removed are sometimes told to take progestagens with their estrogens.

WILL ADDING PROGESTAGEN HELP?

Progestagens, synthetic versions of progesterone, have been used by European gynecologists in conjunction with estrogen replacement for a number of years. Recently they have started to be advocated in this country as well.

Progestagen is most often prescribed for women who have not had hysterectomies who take estrogen-replacement therapy, since it reduces the risk of developing uterine cancer. Advocates of progestagen also recommend it for women who have had hysterectomies to help retard osteoporosis, to help prevent the development of breast cancer, and to normalize the level of endorphins, which are the body's natural painkillers.

But be wary of doctors who assure you that by adding progesterone all the problems of replacement therapy have been solved. They haven't.

In the woman who still retains her uterus, progestagens often result in withdrawal bleeding similar to menstruation. This will not be a consideration for the hysterectomized woman, but the fact that progestagens make some women feel depressed may be. Morrie Gelfand, M.D., of McGill University in Montreal said in a recent symposium, "I have come to the conclusion that adding it may result in such unpleasant side effects that patients refuse to continue taking it." [41]

If you do find you're depressed while taking progestagen, be sure to discuss this with your doctor since changing either the progestagen or its dosage can often help.

Also of concern is what effect progestagens will have on the heart. Most of the progestagens lower the level of high-density lipoprotein cholesterol (HDL cholesterol), the "good" cholesterol that protects against heart attack, and at least some studies have shown that adding progestagens to estrogen nullified the possibly good effects of estrogen on the heart. [42] Addressing this problem in the same round table, Leon Speroff, M.D., chairman of the department of reproductive biology at Case Western Reserve University School of Medicine in Cleveland, Ohio, pointed out that "we don't know the long-term impact of adding progestagens, and we haven't the foggiest idea of what varying the dose will do to the lipids. It's essential that we find an answer soon. More women die of cardiovascular disease than of uterine and breast cancers."

What's more, the doses of progestagens currently being used are much higher than the level normally produced by the body. Dr. García of the University of Pennsylvania Medical School has been using 2.5 milligrams (compared to the 10 milligrams usually prescribed), "but I'm not sure that even that's correct. We're at a very primitive level in terms of just what effect it has on the lining of the uterus. We have even less information about what it does to the breast."

WHAT ABOUT ADDING TESTOSTERONE?

Women who have found their libido diminished following the removal of their ovaries have often found that taking the male hormone testosterone can effectively restore it. This makes sense, since there is evidence that sexual arousal in women is more closely related to testosterone levels than anything else. The two main sources of testosterone in women are the adrenal glands and the ovaries. In some women adrenal production is sufficient, and they do not suffer any loss of libido when their ovaries are removed. Others, however, sense the loss of ovarian testosterone and find that it can be replaced artificially.

Several studies now have shown that testosterone replacement in women not only improves libido and enjoyment of sex but also combats tiredness and lack of concentration. One study showed that libido, measured on a scale of one to 100, increased from an average of 13.5 to 86.1 following testosterone administration.[43]

Other studies have shown that it is testosterone, not estrogen, that improves well-being.[44] Dr. Gelfand, coauthor of one such study, said that adding androgens (of which testosterone is one) to estrogens decreased depression, increased energy and well-being, "and—perhaps unfortunately—appetite as well." He also reported an increase in sexual desire, arousal, and sexual fantasies.[45]

But the side effects of testosterone can be troublesome. You may develop hairiness or mild acne, or your voice may deepen or your clitoris enlarge. If you decide to take testosterone, be sure to be on the lookout for these signs and stop taking it immediately if they should develop.[46]

Many doctors are also concerned that over the long term, testosterone even more than progestagen may increase a woman's risk of heart attack.[47]

The simple truth is that no solution is perfect. Even if you take estrogen, progestagens, and androgens after your ovaries are removed, you still have no assurance that you will feel the same as you felt before the surgery. Hormonally, you won't be the same.[48]

Even if you have no complaints about the effects of the hormones, you may find it a nuisance to have to take pills to replace something that you used to make naturally. "Some women re-sent it," said Dr. García. "Cost may not be the factor. Even the patients who get it at no cost to them still don't like it."

If your menopausal symptoms following hysterectomy or ovarian removal are severe, you may find that treating them so frustrates your physicians that they simply don't want to deal with it. One woman in her late forties who suffered a variety of symptoms following removal of her uterus and ovaries reported that her female gynecologist said to her, "What are you coming to see me for? You don't have any organs!"

Many women, of course, have had this operation and seem to do well enough. Why? Well, as Susanne Morgan, who herself had her uterus and ovaries removed at the age of thirty, said, "Women cope because women are very resilient. But don't trivialize the operation."

Summing Up

Before you agree to a hysterectomy, you should know that it is major surgery that can be followed by a number of complications such as infections and bladder injuries.

But the most common side effects of hysterectomy may be depression, suffered by perhaps half of women under forty, and diminished enjoyment of sex, reported in some studies to occur in about one-third of women.

If your ovaries are also removed, serious medical problems such as osteoporosis are likely to occur if you don't take hormone-replacement therapy. But hormone-replacement therapy has its own problems: besides not always curing the symptoms of ovarian removal, it may cause long-term side effects.

Before you agree to either operation, you should therefore carefully consider whether hysterectomy and ovarian removal are going to help you enough to justify these possible side effects.

Chapter 3

Strategies for Avoiding Hysterectomy

"It is the patient herself who should be in the best position to judge the severity of discomfort and disability, and to decide whether the prospect of future relief is sufficient to justify the immediate costs and risks of hysterectomy." John Bunker, M.D.

"I don't know. I don't know if it was unnecessary. I wasn't there to make a choice or wasn't given the options or the facts. I was asleep." A woman on the Phil Donahue show

A lot of women I know have avoided hysterectomy. How did they do it? Kristie went to a medical library to research alternatives. Mary called the American College of Obstetricians and Gynecologists to find out if hysterectomy was her only option for endometriosis. Monique spoke to other women. Alice changed doctors. I stayed with the same doctor but dug in my heels. Karen cried, at which point her gynecologist described other options.

All of us were told we needed hysterectomies, and all of us found other solutions.

The decision for or against a hysterectomy can be one of the most important decisions you ever make in your life, and you shouldn't make it lightly. But as James Daniell, M.D., a clinical associate professor of gynecology at Vanderbilt University in

Nashville, Tennessee, says, too many women proceed blindly. "People will take their car somewhere and give the car repairman the third degree," he points out, but they're too easily intimidated by a doctor to realize they can ask questions and take their business elsewhere.

We have, of course, been conditioned to be good girls, to believe that doctors have our best interests at heart and that a medical decision is somehow mystical and cannot be made by anyone who hasn't been to medical school. In fact, there is nothing mystical about a medical decision: it should be a rational weighing of the probable risks and benefits of the procedure based on available information. You are just as capable as your doctor of weighing the facts once they are given to you, and you should expect that part of your doctor's job is to set forth the facts in an honest manner.

Don't be intimidated if your doctor tries to hedge by telling you that something is "good medical practice," "indicated," "necessary," or the "treatment of choice." Remember that it was once considered good medical practice to give diethylstilbestrol to pregnant women to prevent miscarriage, even though there was no good evidence that it did so. The drug was later found to cause cancer in daughters born to such women. Remember that it was once thought necessary to tell women they should gain no more than twenty pounds during pregnancy, even though that practice is now thought to have led to smaller, and probably unhealthier, babies. Remember that radical mastectomy was once considered the "treatment of choice" for breast cancer even though there was no good evidence that it was any better than other, less mutilating treatments.

Remember, too, that most hysterectomies are more a quality-of-life than a life-or-death decision. As a result, it's essential that you be an active participant. Your gynecologist may know what disease you have, but he or she probably doesn't know much about your sexuality, your feeling about children, or your feelings about your body—all of which play a very important role in your quality of life. When a gynecologist recommends hysterectomy, he or she is often assuming a great deal, and many of the assumptions may not be correct. Jane, for example, was told by her gynecologist that she didn't want children—based apparently on the fact that she was thirty-three and still using an IUD!

If you are going to be satisfied with your treatment, you must speak up, ask questions, and not be afraid to disagree. The following sections contain some practical information to help you feel more confident as you get more involved.

CHOOSING A DOCTOR

Obviously, technical competence is important. Dr. Daniell suggests asking your doctor questions such as: Are you certified by the American Board of Obstetricians and Gynecologists (i.e., a real specialist)? Where did you get your training? How many of these procedures have you done? Have you written any papers? What's your success rate? Can you ask three satisfied customers to talk to me? You do that automatically, after all, when you want a paint job done on your house.

You are obviously going to be a bit more hesitant if you are your doctor's first patient, or if your doctor is unwilling to give you the names of other patients who have had the procedure. While many good doctors never write papers, those who do are generally considered the experts in the field. In any case, try to determine whether your doctor at least *reads* papers and can relay new information to you logically.

If you're new in the community, try to find out who your family doctor's wife, or your family doctor, goes to herself, or call up the gynecology or operating-room nurse at the local hospital. Both of these are excellent ways to get the names of competent doctors.

If fertility is a consideration, you may wish to consult a fertility specialist before any surgery in order to minimize the chance that the surgery will make it difficult or impossible for you to have children in the future. If you think you might have cancer, consultation with a cancer specialist may allow you to preserve your fertility as well as to survive the cancer.

But technical expertise is not everything. A journalist friend of mine who has reported on medicine for many years says she considers "shared values" the most important quality in a doctor, and I would have to agree with her.

Says Kristie, "The most important thing is to find a doctor who wants to do what you want. Most women, I assume, want to avoid a hysterectomy, so it's important to find a doctor who wants that. Because if you don't, you're constantly fighting someone who thinks you should be doing something different. You don't need that."

Are women doctors any better? One study from Switzerland showed that women who had a female gynecologist were about half as likely to have a hysterectomy as those who had a male gynecologist.[1] Another, in this country, showed that while doctors' wives had a higher rate of hysterectomy than the national average, female doctors themselves had a lower one.[2] But as you will see from the stories in this book, just finding a woman doctor is not a panacea. More important, in my opinion, is finding someone who wants to help you and is willing to listen to you to find out what you want.

Often finding a satisfactory doctor will mean changing from the one you have. This can be hard to do, since women tend to be very loyal to their doctors. But sometimes, said Karyl, "even if you love the guy, you have to move on because he's just not helping you."

RESEARCHING THE ISSUE

As a journalist, I know that I can get much more information during an interview if I have researched the issue in advance. Occasionally I interview someone who is totally forthcoming and able to place issues in their proper perspective. But usually people tell you what *they* think is important, not necessarily what you need to know. Prior research can help you determine the important and controversial issues. If your interviewee tries to evade these, you are in a much better position to get your questions answered.

The same is true of the medical visit. I have found that most doctors will answer questions if you know what to ask. If they won't, you should fire them and find another doctor.

But how do you research a medical issue? Magazines are a common source of medical information and often a good one. But you should be aware of the biases. One is the bias of all journalism to write only about what is new, not necessarily what is important. A bias more specific to the women's magazines is to be upbeat and not to print depressing information, even if it is true. Another is an overreliance on certain medical "experts."

I learned how much weight such "experts" have when I first wrote about fibroids and myomectomy for a women's magazine with a slightly feminist bent. I had no problem being upbeat, since I was very positive about myomectomy. But before the article was printed it was shown to two gynecologists. One kept her comments pretty much to the facts. But the other felt she had a license to make all sorts of value judgments. When I concluded the article saying I would rather have a second myomectomy than a hysterectomy, her comment was: "This woman is unable to deal with her need to have an 'illusion of fertility.' [I was at the time thirty-seven.] She is not acting in a mature fashion. She does not represent the population as a whole—she needs help." In the article I had quoted a gynecologist as saying, "If a woman insisted on a myomectomy, I would honor her request, but depending on her age I would tell her how much I objected. If she was forty-six, I'd tell her she was crazy; if forty-one, perhaps a little less so." The gynecologist commented, "I would not honor her request. If a woman over forty-five refused hysterectomy for fibroids I'd tell her she was crazy. At forty-one she is also stupid."

I pointed out to the editor that this woman was not an expert in myomectomy, while the people I had interviewed were. I also pointed out that the judgments she was making were value judgments, not medical ones, and that despite her comments about my needing help she was not a psychiatrist. Most of my article was published as I had originally written it, and indeed the comments made me so angry I came out even stronger in favor of myomectomy than I had initially. But I learned in the process why so many of the articles on medicine in women's magazines are so watered down.

In my own case I found books to be of little help, since they all reflected the U.S. bias against myomectomy. If you have problems other than fibroids you may find them more helpful. But as I said before, books written by doctors about hysterectomy tend to minimize side effects, while books written by women who have had them may give an abnormally gloomy picture, since women who've had bad experiences with the operation are more likely to write books about it than women who've had good ones. Reading both doctor-written and women-written books may help to put things in perspective.

A somewhat better source of information, if you can gain entrance to a medical library, are articles that appear in the medical journals. You can find the relevant articles either via computer search or the old-fashioned way by looking in the *Index Medicus*, a sort of reader's guide to the medical literature. I have tried to give complete references to the most important articles I have found so that you will be able to look them up for further information if you want. I have also included the subject headings you will need in the glossary on pages 180–83. For example, if you want information on fibroids you must look under the heading "Leiomyomas."

Remember, however, that even the medical literature must be taken with more than a grain of salt because it is riddled with opinions. You need to look up a number of different articles on the subject to get a balanced picture. A particularly good single source of information is a magazine called *Contemporary Ob/Gyn*. Here, experts from around the country are invited to participate in panel discussions on topics of interest, and you are privy to the differences of opinion that some of the better U.S. gynecologists may have. The magazine is much more informative than the women's magazines, but it is much more clearly written than most of the journals.

Support groups, both formal and informal, are also excellent sources of information. The Endometriosis Association, for example, not only gives emotional support but is also an unbeatable source of information about the disease and a way to find out which doctors are doing what. You should talk to other women informally, too, particularly if you can find women you respect who have had the same problems you are having. In my own case, I found that women who had never had fibroids, particularly those who didn't know what they were, were often freaked out by the word "tumor." Talking to other women with fibroids was much more helpful. While we didn't always have the same symptoms, or choose the same solutions, sharing our experiences was nevertheless worthwhile.

MAKING A LIST

Some doctors ridicule patients who bring a list of questions with them to a consultation. The French even have a name for such patients, *les malades des petits papiers* ("patients with little papers"). The rationale for such ridicule is that if you need a note to remind you of something, it can't be that important. This, of course, is ridiculous. Most people write lists all the time to go to the grocery store, plan a dinner party, chair a meeting, conduct an interview, or plan a schedule.

Most doctors I have observed during sixteen years of covering medical meetings have either notes or an entire text before them when they give a presentation (and those who don't often should), and I do not take this to mean that they don't know what they are saying.

Upon learning that her cone biopsy (a minor surgical operation in which a slice of the cervix is removed) had shown invasive cervical cancer, Maureen looked up a friend who had worked in a pathology lab.

Together they looked through a lot of medical books and decided that invasive cervical cancer was one definite case where hysterectomy was justified.

Her friend told her to make a list of anything she wanted to know, even such things as "What can I eat after the operation?" She wrote her doctor a long letter full of questions like, "Will I have tubes up my nose? What kind of anesthesia will you use? What kind of painkiller will you give me? How long will I be in the hospital? What will I be able to do afterward? What precisely are you going to do? Will I keep my ovaries?" She subsequently met with the doctor for forty-five minutes and asked him the questions in person, which allowed her to go into surgery with a much greater degree of reassurance. In fact, she found that the worst part of the experience was the gas pains, which nobody had warned her about.

OBTAINING RECORDS

In France, all copies of medical lab reports, Pap smears, operative reports, and x-rays are sent directly to the patient as well as the doctor. As a result, I am able to provide my doctors in the United States with a thorough report of everything my doctors found in France.

I hope that such a practice soon becomes standard in the United States. While I didn't always understand the detailed French pathology report on the Pap smear, I nevertheless felt much better about having it than I do about the little cards I now receive telling me no malignant cells were found, since the Pap is really testing for premalignant cells anyway. As you will see in subsequent chapters, in many cases women have not been told their diagnosis or that their uterus was perforated, say, during a D & C. Getting a video of your laser surgery, as some endometriosis patients are now doing, seems a bit strange at first, but upon reflection I like the idea more and more.

Maureen asked for her pathology reports when told she had cancer. Her doctor was originally reluctant to give them to her, but she said,

"I'm not going to publish them in the newspaper. I can understand most of it because I had Latin in high school. What I don't understand I can look up. I'm not going to get hysterical. It's my information, and I want to know what's been said."

The pathology report proved very helpful, she said, because she was able to get a second opinion over the phone. Her surgeon was prominent in the field, and her pathologist well known, so after hearing what was on the path report, the second doctor suggested that there was really no need for another opinion. She went ahead with her radical hysterectomy, reassured that her doctor was not performing it without good reason.

SECOND OPINIONS

By all means get a second opinion. Dr. Winston's statement—that 90 percent of the women he sees who have been recommended for hysterectomy have little or no pathology—should be an eye-opener.

If the doctor gets mad when you suggest getting a second opinion, Dr. Daniell says you should immediately walk out because if a doctor is so insecure about a second opinion you probably don't want him operating on you anyway. "I have confidence in my opinion, and if a patient gets another opinion from somebody else I'm sure it will be the same as mine, or at least I'll be able to defend mine to my satisfaction. If the doctor's upset about the idea of a second opinion, then there's something wrong with him," he says. A poll of doctors by *M.D.* magazine found that over half agreed with the statement "I would never have elective surgery unless I got a second opinion." [3]

But even if the second opinion agrees with the first, make sure you understand exactly what will be done and the reasons for it, and make sure you agree with them. "There are so many women who answer 'I don't know' when I ask them what they had done," says Dr. Daniell. "American women have refused to be assertive too long."

Be sure you understand whether hysterectomy, or any other procedure, is being recommended because you run the risk of dying if it is not performed. Can irreversible damage result if you don't have a hysterectomy now? Is there any danger in waiting awhile? Is the hysterectomy only being recommended to cure the symptoms you have told your doctors about? In that case, are the symptoms bothering *you* enough to justify hysterectomy? And what are the alternatives?

PAYING THE BILL

Many women have problems being straightforward when asking about money, and where doctors are concerned we're all too inclined to pay what's asked without shopping around. While I'm very assertive about getting my medical questions answered, when it comes to money I become as blindly obedient as anyone. Maureen wasn't, and I think her story illustrates why none of us should be.

When Maureen asked how much her radical hysterectomy would cost, she was told by the secretary $7,500. "I said, 'Oh, my insurance company will pay,' and the secretary said, 'No, the insurance won't cover it.' It turned out the going rate was about $3,000. I called several doctors to find out what their rates were, and found $7,500 was way out of line. I called my surgeon back and told him, if that is indeed your fee, I can't afford it. He then gave me the other secretary, who said that they would take whatever the insurance paid. It didn't make me question my doctor's skill as a surgeon, because I knew he had one of the top reputations in the country, but it made me feel kind of bad. My insurance company told me they wish more patients would do this."

CONSENT TO TREATMENT

Most of us are familiar with the consent forms brought around in hospitals for us to sign the night before surgery. This in fact is not a valid consent, and probably would not hold up in court if there was no evidence that we had actually discussed the treatment with our doctor, says Fay Rozovsky, a lawyer and public health specialist who is also the author of *Consent to Treatment: A Practical Guide* (Little, Brown and Company). "Consent forms have unfortunately come to supplant the consent process in many institutions. People refer to it as the consent. It is not the consent. By coming to rely on these forms, people are forgetting to talk to one another."

"Consent is a process, it's a dialogue of exchange of information," says Dr. Rozovsky. The law, she explains, requires that before surgery, patients be given significant information regarding probable risks and benefits, together with information on the availability of reasonable alternative forms of treatment (for example, treatment with drugs or a less radical surgical intervention) and the risks and benefits associated with these alternatives. The risk of forgoing treatment at all should also be discussed. The doctor should answer any questions the patient has in a manner the patient can understand. The response should be candid and to the point.

Let me give you an example of how the consent process can work in recounting in my own experiences in France and America.

> *When my French surgeon said, "We must operate," without any further clarification except that the operation would be to remove my grapefruit-sized fibroid, I asked him, "What do I risk if I refuse?" "You are still young and could have children," he told me. "If we don't take out the fibroid now, you may have to have a hysterectomy later."*

This exchange illustrates one feature of the consent process: finding out the consequences of no treatment at all. It also illustrates, I think, that doctors often don't volunteer such information but will answer if you ask them questions outright. This surgeon spoke to me with such urgency that I often wonder whether his other patients believe myomectomy is necessary to save their lives. Because I asked, I was able to place the surgery in a different perspective.

· · ·

Although I liked this surgeon, I found another because I didn't like the high-handed way I was treated by the secretary of the gynecology department at his hospital. My second surgeon was not as sure as the first that he would be able to take out the fibroid without the uterus. Upon seeing my downcast face, he then made the following proposition: If upon opening the abdomen he found he could not remove the fibroid, he would not remove anything at all. I would thus retain some chance, albeit small, of eventually having children. I agreed. This agreement has shocked a number of doctors and others who believe that "if you open her up, you've got to take something out." But I opted for the operation to safeguard my fertility, not because I was suffering in any way. If I had lost my fertility altogether, I would have been in worse shape than before the operation; if I simply was sewn back up, all I would have lost was the recuperation time from surgery.

This illustrates another feature of the consent process: agreeing on priorities in case something unexpected arises. You cannot ask your surgeon to do something technically impossible, but you and he can agree on where to go if he finds something unexpected such as fibroids that cannot be removed, or cancer, or if you begin to bleed excessively during the operation.

My French surgeon wanted to do the operation via a bikini or Pfannenstiel incision, and I initially resisted. I had been brought up in the U.S. Bible Belt, where aesthetics are not taken nearly as seriously as they are in France. I believed at the time that appearance was not an important enough consideration to influence the choice of incision. He then told me that the bikini incision was also stronger, which I found more convincing. In the end, I was very happy with the incision, which was completely hidden in the pubic hair, and requested another for my second myomectomy.

The surgeon, in other words, is not always wrong!

When I found out my fibroids had started growing back, on my return to the United States I sought out a surgeon I had interviewed for a magazine article on fibroids. I knew he used the laser for myomecto-

mies, but I chose him because he had been the only one I'd interviewed in my area who had given any weight to emotional factors in the decision to opt for myomectomy. By this time I was thirty-seven.
He recommended hysterectomy on the basis that only one myomectomy could be done. This I knew to be an opinion, not a fact. The uterus does not disintegrate after a second myomectomy, although with every operation there is a risk of scar tissue forming.
I refused.

This illustrates another facet of the consent process: you always have the right to refuse medical treatment, even though such treatment may be felt by the doctor to be in your best interest.

He then suggested that we watch and wait, and I came in every six months for checkups. Shortly after my thirty-ninth birthday, he found fibroids were making my uterus the size of a five-month pregnancy. If I still wanted to avoid hysterectomy, he said, now was the time to operate. But he told me to think seriously about whether or not I wanted another myomectomy. I wrote him a long letter explaining why I did.

The letter was to protect both me and my surgeon. I feel strongly that if one goes against medical advice, one should take the responsibility for any untoward consequences that result from that decision. Had I died or become brain-damaged during the second myomectomy, my family might have sued, and since the general opinion in this country seems to be that two myomectomies are unjustified, my doctor might have been in a bad position (although I could have just as readily died or been brain-damaged during a hysterectomy). The letter provided a degree of legal protection for him at the same time that it showed him I had thought about the issue myself.
Dr. Rozovsky says that while in most cases such a letter is not necessary, there is a tendency across North America for patients to give their doctors documents such as letters or living wills that specify they should not be kept alive on machines if they are brain-dead. She suggests that a letter may be a good idea

if you are afraid the doctor may want to remove more than you want removed. There is no need to have the letter notarized, she says.

"You realize you might have to have further surgery later," my U.S. surgeon said. I said, yes, I thought this a small price to pay. I also told him I thought removing an organ to prevent further problems with it was similar to committing suicide to prevent further problems with the body in general.

Technically, my surgeon was correct in pointing out the disadvantages of myomectomy. He did not, however, point out any disadvantages of hysterectomy, although there are many, as you have seen.

"I'm not sure I can remove all the fibroids," he said.

I then told him of my French doctor's offer to sew me back up if he couldn't perform the myomectomy. My American doctor and I knew from the sonogram that this time I had many small fibroids rather than one large one. Couldn't he just remove as many as he could and leave the rest? Since it is usually the size of fibroids, not their presence, that causes problems, this seemed reasonable to me.

He said he didn't like to perform an incomplete operation.

I told him that perhaps he didn't like to but that this seemed to be the best option for me.

He then promised under no circumstances to perform a hysterectomy, adding, however, that he thought I was crazy. He then added, "Women drive me crazy."

I suggested perhaps he ought to change specialties.

He nodded.

The second myomectomy, at least for me, was easy compared to the negotiation I had to go through to get it. All the same, my experience shows that even if you cannot find the perfect doctor, you may be able to work with one of good faith. Keep in mind that anything done to you should be for your benefit and that often you must help the doctor decide what that is.

What's the bottom line, then? Besides finding a technically competent doctor, you must get one who is willing to use the best treatment for you among possible treatments for your disease. Always keep uppermost in your mind that you should never submit to a treatment unless you are convinced it is the best among your possible choices; remember also that you must play an active role in making this decision.

C h a p t e r 4

Fibroids—the Most Common Reason Women Are Told They Need a Hysterectomy

Fibroid tumors are the most common reason doctors recommend hysterectomy in the United States, accounting for some 30 to 50 percent of all hysterectomies.[1] About 20 to 30 percent of women have fibroids, and in autopsy studies, some 50 percent have been found to have evidence of fibroids.[2]

In fact, fibroids are so common that many physicians consider them boring.

While the annual meetings of the American College of Obstetricians and Gynecologists usually have multiple sessions devoted to endometriosis, pain, and dysfunctional bleeding, not a single session was devoted to fibroids in 1985, and in 1986 only one was. "Why don't you write about endometriosis?" asked one gynecologist when I was interviewing him about an article on fibroid tumors. "Now *that's* really a horrible disease." An editorialist in *Obstetrical and Gynecological Survey* called fibroids "not of great interest to investigators."[3]

This lack of interest undoubtedly has slowed any progress in medical treatments for fibroids. In addition, it has tended to suppress information about treatments that have been available for years. For while there are no magical cures, there are alternatives that may be much more acceptable to you than hysterectomy.

> *Karen, an educational administrator, started to have pains in the lower part of her abdomen when she was about twenty-eight, and a fibroid tumor of the uterus was eventually diagnosed. About seven years later, the pains became "so excruciating that they would wake me up in the middle of the night," she said. When she went to the gynecologist, he told her, "Your uterus is all out of whack," and said she would probably have to have a hysterectomy.*
>
> *"My first reaction," said Karen, who is single, "was to cry. Then he talked about the alternative. He told me about myomectomy." Karen had the myomectomy and knew as soon as she recovered from the anesthesia that it had eliminated the pain from her fibroid.*

Myomectomy, or the removal of fibroids while preserving the uterus, is one alternative. Most of the time myomectomy is major surgery, but sometimes the fibroids can be removed through the vagina in a procedure known as hysteroscopic myomectomy (see page 183). Doing nothing is another alternative, often quite effective. And while currently there are no good medications for fibroids, very recently several centers have started experimenting with drugs known as GnRH analogs that can sometimes shrink fibroids dramatically. So far, GnRH analogs have a number of problems. But if further development can iron them out, "we may be put out of business doing surgery for fibroids," said Dr. Hutchins.

WHAT ARE FIBROIDS?

Gynecologists don't particularly like the name "fibroids" because it implies that the tumors arise out of fibrous tissue, which they don't. They prefer the terms "leiomyomas," or more simply "myomas," since these tumors arise in the myometrium (muscular layer of the uterus). The myometrium lies underneath the part that actually bleeds each month, the endometrium. I will continue to use the term "fibroids," however. Very few of us talk about our leiomyomas or even our myomas; we talk about our fibroids.

Depending on their location, fibroids are referred to as submucous, intramural, or subserous. Submucous fibroids grow on the inside of the uterus, subserous ones on the outside, and intramural ones within the uterine wall. The difference can be important. In general, subserous and intramural fibroids must be relatively large to cause any problems, while submucous fibroids —those on the inside—can cause heavy bleeding and fertility problems even when they are small.[4]

Each fibroid is thought to be derived from a single cell. All the cells in a given fibroid are identical to each other, but they are not identical to cells in other fibroids, even in the same uterus.[5]

Fibroids differ from normal myometrial tissue in that they are more responsive to estrogen.[6] This probably explains why they tend to grow during the years in which a woman's ovaries are producing estrogen and to shrink at menopause and during the artificial menopause induced by the GnRH analogs. It probably also explains at least part of the bleeding abnormalities produced by fibroids that are explained on page 59.

An inherited tendency to fibroids seems to exist. They are about nine times more frequent in black women than in white women, and they tend to run in families.[7] But I have also read that they tend to run among friends—in other words, that perhaps diet or life-style is as important. In my own experience, my mother, myself, and several of my best friends, who come from a variety of ethnic backgrounds, have had some type of surgery for fibroids. They are just very, very common, no matter what your origins.

For a long time doctors suspected that fibroids were more common in women who hadn't had children, and recently it has been shown that the more children you have, the less likely you are to have fibroids. The birth-control pill may protect somewhat against fibroids,[8] as does smoking. The more you weigh, the more likely you are to have fibroids. Women who weigh less than 55 kilograms (120 pounds) have a particularly low risk, and the risk rises by 21 percent for each 10 kilograms (22 pounds) of weight. All these findings tend to support the theory that estrogen stimulation unopposed by progesterone will cause fibroids to grow. Pregnancy and birth-control pills tend to give the body high levels of progestagen in relation to estrogen, and smoking tends to reduce estrogen levels while increased body fat increases estrogen levels.

Can any of these facts be translated into preventive measures? Well, from a practical point of view, it probably makes sense to try to keep your weight down if you know you have fibroids or that someone in your family did. It might also make sense to take the birth-control pill, although this recommendation is controversial, particularly as some doctors fear that at least in certain women the pill can cause growth of fibroids.[9] Obviously, smoking as a way to cut down on the estrogen your body produces is no solution at all, since it causes a host of other, more serious problems. Having lots of children, meanwhile, should be seen as a solution only if you want them.

WATCHING AND WAITING

Most serious gynecologists would agree that small fibroids that are causing no symptoms need no treatment whatsoever. Even doctors prone to operate would not consider a hysterectomy for fibroids legitimate unless the uterus was at least the size of a three-month pregnancy or greater.

Many gynecologists, however, apparently do recommend hysterectomy for such small fibroids. Edward E. Wallach, M.D., professor of obstetrics and gynecology at the University of Pennsylvania School of Medicine, says, "I am amazed at the number of patients without symptoms and with perhaps only the slightest irregularity or enlargement of the uterus who are told their fibroids need removal."[10]

You may be alarmed by the word "tumor," but fibroids are

benign tumors: they do not invade other organs, although they sometimes grow large enough to put pressure on them. There is a small chance—about 1 in 200—that a fibroid may contain a malignant tumor known as a leiomyosarcoma. If the fibroid is growing rapidly, the chances of malignancy are greater, but even in these cases the chances are small. As Dr. Hutchins points out, most fibroids grow in spurts, increasing rapidly in size for a while and then lying dormant. If your gynecologist thinks that your fibroids are growing rapidly, it may simply be that she has examined you just after a spurt of growth.

At just what size fibroids should be treated at all is matter of judgment, and gynecologists differ in their recommendations. While the three-month pregnancy size is generally a lower limit, fibroids can get enormous without causing debilitating symptoms. Dr. J. A. Chalmers, an English gynecologist, recounts his experience with a forty-nine-year-old member of the women's Royal Air Force who so destroyed the symmetry of the parade on one occasion that she was thought by her commanding officer to be pregnant. She was exonerated only when her protuberance was found to be a twenty-four-pound fibroid.[11]

"How many women have been shown to develop clinical problems because of a twelve-week-size uterus?" Dr. Hutchins rhetorically asked a session he gave at the 1986 meeting of the American College of Obstetricians and Gynecologists. "My experience is, not very many. I think we've all seen women in our practices who have monstrous-sized uteri and are asymptomatic. They just have this enormous tumor which is very impressive and should go into the Guinness book of records. And in fact they're doing quite well."

Dr. Hutchins said he did not know of any data where large numbers of women with untreated fibroids were followed to find out what the incidence of complications actually is.

Susan, an office worker in her mid-forties, has a fibroid uterus the size of a twenty-four-week pregnancy. Nearly every doctor she has seen has "read me the riot act about this humongous thing growing inside me. Repeatedly I've been told, warned, urged of the dire consequences of this enlarging fibroid uterus. It has been the kind of attitude where they want to sign me in tomorrow for a hysterectomy. I've had it for nine years, and I'm very, very happy that I haven't rushed into a hysterectomy."

Susan had some bleeding problems, particularly right after her IUD was removed, and became anemic, but her anemia was easily treated with iron supplements. Eventually her periods became lighter. *"I think that if the alternative is surgery or wearing skirts rather than slacks during your period, the choice is pretty clear."*

Susan has no particular problems from her fibroids now except that they make her abdomen bulge. If she made a mistake, it was in not having a myomectomy, since she has been told it would be impossible now. But unless her fibroids begin causing more symptoms than they are now, she sees no reason to go for surgery.

SYMPTOMS THAT CAN BE CAUSED BY FIBROIDS

Depending upon their position and size, fibroids can cause various symptoms, estimated to occur in 25 to 50 percent of women known to have fibroids.[12] These are:

Bleeding. Fibroids can cause both heavy bleeding during periods and irregular bleeding between periods. There are several reasons for this.[13] For one thing, fibroids tend to enlarge the uterus in general and the endometrium in particular, providing a greater surface area to bleed each month. For another, fibroids can push against the blood vessels in the uterus, distorting their normal flow. Still a third way that fibroids may distort the normal bleeding pattern is to create local areas of hyperplasia, or areas that have become overly stimulated by estrogen (see chapter 5). Since fibroids are more receptive to estrogen than to progesterone,[14] the normal balance between the two hormones is altered, and since estrogen tends to increase bleeding and progesterone to keep it in check, the balance is tipped in favor of heavier bleeding. According to Dr. Hutchins, abnormal bleeding occurs in approximately one-third of women with fibroid tumors.

.   .   .

Pressure Symptoms. Because fibroids can grow large, they can push against other organs such as the bladder and bowel. In most cases, said Dr. Hutchins, the symptoms are not that serious. While minor symptoms such as needing to urinate frequently are relatively common in women with fibroids, he said, "frank urinary obstruction and overt urinary tract disease is relatively rare." While it seems difficult to determine the actual incidence of such disease, in a study from Benin, Nigeria, reporting 180 cases of fibroids serious enough to be hospitalized, only 6 patients complained of urinary frequency and another 6 had urinary retention.[15]

While writing this book, a friend of a friend telephoned me to say that she had just seen a new gynecologist, who told her that she had fibroids and should have a hysterectomy since they could damage her urinary tract. Her former gynecologist had seen no reason for a hysterectomy. She had no symptoms and did not want a hysterectomy. But the gynecologist had worried her: she did not want to end up with damaged kidneys a few years down the road. What should she do?

I tried to determine just what such a woman, with no symptoms, risked by refusing a hysterectomy. Since I was not a doctor and had not examined her, could it be possible that the fibroids in her particular case were in a position where they would suddenly cause kidney damage? I called Dr. Winston, whom I knew was not hysterectomy-happy, to ask his opinion.

It's true, he said, that if fibroids are large and extend out to the sides, they can put pressure on the ureters, the tubes carrying urine from the kidney to the bladder. But the fact that this *might* happen, he said, is not a reason to perform a hysterectomy, although it is a reason perhaps to order certain tests such as renal sonograms or IVPs (intravenous pyelograms) from time to time to see if in fact the fibroid is pushing on the ureters. Surgery isn't necessary until there is already an impingement on the ureters.

Serious bowel obstruction is considered even rarer.

Many women just feel full. If you complain of such fullness, your doctor may begin talking of "pressure symptoms," an ominous-sounding term that must be taken with a grain of salt, I found.

About five years after my first myomectomy, my uterus had again grown back to the size of a twenty-week pregnancy with multiple fibroids. My gynecologist was most disturbed by the fact that he could no longer feel my ovaries, which didn't particularly disturb me since I have never had any ovarian problems. He asked me if I had any symptoms, and I told him my periods were heavy, with a particularly heavy spurt occurring for a brief period during the fourth, fifth, or sixth day that could soak a super tampon in ten or fifteen minutes. I had also been told by the blood donation center that I was anemic, with a hemoglobin of 9.5, and although this made me ineligible as a blood donor, they said it was probably not that serious for my health and advised me to take Geritol. I'm sure I minimized my symptoms to some degree because I did not want to give my gynecologist an excuse for performing a hysterectomy.

I also mentioned that I could tell my skirts were fitting tighter, and he nodded and said, "Ah, pressure symptoms," and wrote it down. My feeling at the time was, "So this is what 'pressure symptoms' means." I had always assumed that the term stood for something more ominous than tight waistbands, that it probably meant my internal organs were being dangerously crammed together. Had my gynecologist not used the term then, in conjunction with my tight skirts, but had later told me hysterectomy was justified because I had pressure symptoms, I would have been somewhat frightened, and perhaps more willing to consent.

My subsequent myomectomy, in which some forty fibroids were removed and my uterus reduced from a twenty-week size to about a ten-week size, significantly reduced my periods, eliminating the heavy spurt, and with it the anemia. It didn't, however, eliminate the "pressure symptoms" because I gained weight in the recovery period and my skirts became even tighter than before. Luckily, from my point of view the pressure symptoms were not at all the main reason for agreeing to surgery and so I was not unhappy that they had not been cured.

. . .

Infertility. Fibroids may cause infertility, but most infertility experts usually recommend ruling out other causes of infertility before anything is done about the fibroids. However, Veasy C. Buttram, Jr., M.D., a professor in the division of endocrinology-fertility at Baylor College of Medicine in Houston, Texas, points out that fibroids may be more important as a cause of infertility in black women. In his patients treated for infertility, he found that fibroids were the sole cause of infertility in 9.1 percent of black patients but in only 1.8 percent of white patients.[16] Fibroids can also increase the risk of spontaneous abortion, probably from uterine irritability and contractility, and may complicate pregnancy in other ways. They may also make delivery by cesarean section advisable.

WILL HYSTERECTOMY CURE FIBROIDS?

Obviously, the answer is yes, and it should relieve your symptoms if they are due to fibroids. Heavy and abnormal bleeding will definitely cease, as should any pressure symptoms if they are really due to fibroids. A friend whose nine-pound uterus was removed told me she should have had the operation sooner because she had been miserable before. Another friend who'd had a myomectomy and then a hysterectomy said she should have had the hysterectomy in the first place. But if you would rather preserve your uterus, read on.

MYOMECTOMY AS AN ALTERNATIVE

Myomectomy means removal of the myoma or myomas. Usually, if you have only a few fibroids, it is a relatively easy operation that practically any gynecologist ought to be able to do. If you have more than a few fibroids, your gynecologist may say that myomectomy is impossible. This may not be true; often what it means is that it is impossible for that particular gynecologist.

Surgeons who have taken an interest in myomectomy are almost always able to perform the operation.

Dr. Victor Bonney, for example, an English gynecologist who popularized myomectomy in the early part of this century, once removed 225 fibroids from a single uterus, many years before technological innovations such as the laser. His mortality rate was between 1 and 2 percent, similar to the mortality rate for hysterectomy at that time.[17] Dr. Bonney wrote in 1931, "Today it may be said that it is unusual to meet with a case of fibroids—no matter how numerous the tumours, how large or how placed—that is beyond the scope of conservative surgery." The size of the fibroids didn't stop Dr. Bonney either: "I have performed multiple myomectomy in cases where the total mass was about that of a full-term pregnancy."[18] Dr. Winston told me that the largest number he has personally removed is 60 or 80, and that he very frequently removes 16 to 20

Many gynecologists require that you agree to a hysterectomy if you are to undergo myomectomy in case the myomectomy proves impossible to perform. "Impossible," of course, is a relative term. To some surgeons, this agreement means that if you start bleeding uncontrollably and the only way to stop the bleeding is to perform a hysterectomy, they have that permission. To others, it means that if cancer is found they will remove the uterus and ovaries then and there to save you a further operation. To others it means that they cannot remove all the fibroids. To still others, it means that the myomectomy will be more difficult than they thought and they prefer to perform the easier hysterectomy.

I asked some surgeons skilled in performing myomectomies how often they had to perform unexpected hysterectomies during myomectomies, and they said very rarely. For example, Alan Berkeley, M.D., at New York Hospital said it was true in his experience only when cancer was unexpectedly found. Be sure to ask your doctor how many myomectomies he or she has turned into hysterectomies. Also be sure to ask what would make him perform a hysterectomy, and make sure you agree with the reasons. I'm certain, for example, that had I not made it perfectly clear that I would accept hysterectomy only if I risked dying otherwise, my surgeon would have performed one when he first saw my uterus, which he described as "a disaster."

WILL MYOMECTOMY CURE THE SYMPTOMS?

Dr. Buttram reviewed the cases of a number of published studies on myomectomy and found that 81 percent of patients with heavy bleeding reported a reduction or resolution of this problem following myomectomy. In women whose spontaneous abortions were due to fibroids, their 41 percent abortion rate before myomectomy was reduced to 19 percent postoperatively, which is not too much higher than the 10 percent rate in the general population. In infertile patients in whom all other causes of infertility had been ruled out, 54 percent conceived postoperatively.[19]

Dr. Buttram believes that chances of successful conception tend to be better if the uterus has not grown too large when the myomectomy is performed. For this reason, he recommends considering myomectomy if you have large fibroids and eventually wish to conceive. "For the patient who wishes to delay conception for a year or longer and has a myomatous uterus of ten to twelve weeks gestational size or larger, or one that is rapidly growing, myomectomy is recommended for several reasons." The larger and more numerous the tumors, the greater the difficulty in removing them through a single incision. In addition, the risk of complications such as blood loss, development of postoperative adhesions, and damage to the uterus is greater when myomectomy is performed on a larger uterus. Such complications may ultimately compromise fertility. If you delay myomectomy, he wrote, you may allow the tumors to reach a size where myomectomy is no longer possible.

On the down side, adhesions caused by the operation may themselves compromise fertility. Your best bet if you have large fibroids would probably be to consult with a fertility specialist if you feel you may wish to become pregnant later. As we shall see, fertility specialists are also a good choice to perform myomectomy, since they are familiar with microsurgical techniques that can minimize adhesions.

Jessica, a geologist, was nearing thirty-five when her gynecologist recommended that she have a myomectomy because he felt if her fibroids got larger they would so weaken the uterine wall that the operation wouldn't be successful.

She had the myomectomy. An infection prolonged her hospital stay to a total of six days, and her recovery was somewhat like that of women who have had c-sections. She was on disability for a total of six weeks. While she had most of her strength back after a month, "It took quite a while before I could do things like sit-ups again." It took about a year for her abdominal strength to return to normal.

Her periods are less heavy now, "thank goodness." Jessica, who has gotten married since her myomectomy, said that she has never had a child or tried to get pregnant. "I'm kind of putting off the decision, and one of these years I'll have to decide once and for all."

If she had it to do over, would she still choose to have a myomectomy? "Oh, absolutely. I don't like the idea of needlessly removing body organs, irrespective of the issue of whether you want to have kids or not." While her fibroids have not recurred, she thinks she would probably opt for another myomectomy if they did.

THE DISADVANTAGES OF MYOMECTOMY

Recurrence. My own case illustrates one of the disadvantages of myomectomy: recurrence. Myomectomy is not, to use that favorite term of gynecologists, "definitive," and as long as you have a uterus, you can get fibroids. I am always puzzled, however, at the importance gynecologists give to the issue of recurrence. Yes, it can happen, and it does in about 10 to 20 percent of myomectomized women.[20] Yes, the patient should be told that it can happen. But while I would have preferred that my fibroids not recur, I have no regrets about either the first or the second myomectomy. If they recur again, my own choice would either be to do nothing at all or to have a third myomectomy, although I undoubtedly would have some trouble finding a gynecologist willing to do a third. I might have to go back to France.

But while I find that even a 20 percent recurrence rate doesn't seem to be that strong a disadvantage to myomectomy, there is some evidence that the rate would be lower if the operation were performed thoroughly the first time. The risk of recurrence is also probably less the older you are.

Both these assertions have their basis in the work of Victor Bonney. Bonney advocated an extremely thorough examination of the entire uterus during the operation, with even tiny seedling tumors located and removed. Bonney's recurrence rate was 2.3 percent, and the women who did have recurrences tended to be the younger women.

Bonney wrote in 1931, "My experience leads me to believe that the tendency to the formation of these tumors is a passing phase in the uterine tissues and not a continuous defect. . . . I believe that in most instances the nuclei of all the fibroids a woman is ever going to grow are laid down by the time she has reached 30 years of age, or but very little over."[21]

If myomectomy is performed after the age of thirty-five, then, the surgeon is likely to be able to see all the fibroids and remove them. In younger women, some of the fibroids may be too tiny to see at surgery, and may therefore grow back a few years later.

"It is just in these exceptionally young patients that the desirability of saving the uterus is greatest," Bonney wrote, "and if surgery can restore their [fertility] for even a few years, or, better still, enable them to have even one child, no inconsiderable gain is effected."

Since Bonney's paper was published fifty years ago, I asked several gynecologists if his observations had been superseded by later studies. "No one in the world has had his kind of experience," Dr. Winston said, suggesting that gynecologists who have the higher recurrence rates are not doing the Bonney procedure. His own rate of recurrence, he said, is much lower than 15 percent.

"Bonney searched them out to the nth degree," said Dr. García. "Interestingly, this guy showed the lowest need for repeat surgery. The more meticulous you are about trying to find the small seedlings, the better it is from the point of view of recurrence."

Dr. García agrees with Bonney that older women have fewer recurrences. As a result, he is willing to consider myomectomy for women too old to have children. "I think there is an open-book controversy about how old the individual should be as to when one should recommend a hysterectomy as opposed to a myomectomy. I don't think that's a closed chapter because I don't think we know enough about the value of the cervix and uterus to the individual in terms of her sexuality."

Adhesions. Any surgery may cause the formation of adhesions, or scar tissue that sticks together, but myomectomy seems to be particularly likely to. "Myomectomies are one of the major operations that cause adhesions," said Jay Schinfeld, M.D., an associate professor of obstetrics and gynecology at Temple University and chief of endocrine infertility at Abington Memorial Hospital in Philadelphia.

Some individuals tend to form adhesions more readily than others, just as some individuals form keloids much more readily than others. Adhesions may lead to infertility and sometimes to chronic pain; in any case, they tend to make each repeat surgery more difficult.

Dr. Schinfeld said that there is no surefire way to prevent adhesions altogether, but so-called microsurgical techniques have been shown to damage tissues less. "Microsurgical technique doesn't necessarily mean using the microscope itself," he said. Rather, it means using needles, sutures, and other surgical materials that cause a minimum of tissue damage and using fingers rather than instruments. Since blood contains a substance known as fibrin that is inflammatory and can cause adhesions to form, surgeons versed in microsurgical technique will attempt "to be absolutely immaculate in terms of controlling bleeding so that there's absolutely not one drop of blood." He said that while it was originally thought that the laser would decrease adhesion formation, so far this has not been shown.

A woman's best chance of decreasing adhesions during myomectomy, he said, is "finding someone who's done many of them, who can do them quickly and minimize the bleeding."

Do most gynecologists practice microsurgical technique to prevent adhesions? "It's not a common practice in gynecologic surgery," Dr. García said. "Infertility surgeons would do this as a matter of course. A woman would be better served finding an infertility surgeon if she wants a myomectomy than by asking her local gynecologist to do it. She might get a list of the Society of Reproductive Surgeons within the American Fertility Society. It's not all-inclusive, but at least it's a start for her." (See page 188 for the address of the American Fertility Society.)

Blood loss. Another objection gynecologists have to myomectomy is that it causes more blood loss than hysterectomy. While this is true, a variety of techniques can be used to cut down on bleeding. Dr. García uses a tourniquet technique. Some physicians use the chemical pitressin, which cuts blood loss but in large quantities can provoke hypertensive crises during surgery. Dr. Buttram believes that using a vertical midline incision can cut blood loss by restricting the incision to the least vascular part of the uterus. Some gynecologists like to use the laser to control blood loss. David McLaughlin, M.D., an assistant clinical professor of obstetrics and gynecology at Wright State University Medical School in Dayton, Ohio, found that the average blood loss for patients undergoing conventional myomectomy was 311 milliliters per patient and for those undergoing laser myomectomy 200 milliliters per patient.[22]

IS A LASER MYOMECTOMY BETTER?

Perhaps because of our love of technology, we may tend to consider the laser magic rather than a surgical tool that might or might not give somewhat better results. Many people, for example, don't realize that a laser is often just another way of cutting, and that even with a laser myomectomy the abdomen must be cut open, either by laser or by a scalpel.

My first myomectomy was done with a conventional scalpel; my second was done by laser. Did it make a difference?

Perhaps, in two ways. During the first operation I was given two units of blood and in the second I wasn't given any blood, even though the second was a much more extensive procedure that involved entering the uterine cavity. This difference might have been due to the laser's ability to control blood loss, but it might equally have been due to the fact that the first procedure was done in France prior to the AIDS scare. Blood has not been particularly scarce in France, and since it is mostly provided by volunteers, not paid donors who are more likely to be drug addicts, the risk of hepatitis is low. The French surgeon may simply have felt there was no reason not to give blood.

The second difference had to do with the amount of pain I experienced. In neither case did I have much pain in the days following my surgery, and I didn't require any medication at all twenty-four hours after surgery. I did have considerable pain the day of my nonlaser myomectomy. The lessened pain the second time around may have been due to the laser, but it may also have been due either to the type of incision I had or the way I was given painkillers. I had a bikini incision the first time, a midline the second, and the bikini, while ultimately stronger as well as prettier, supposedly produces more postoperative pain. The first time around, painkillers were given only when I asked for them; the second, they were offered at regular intervals, which is a more efficient way of controlling pain.

The most important benefit of the laser to the patient, in my opinion, is that if the doctor likes to use it he or she is more likely to persist and do the meticulous operating that a myomectomy requires. I would therefore not choose my surgeon for a myomectomy solely on the basis of whether he or she uses a laser. Much more important, I feel, is the surgeon's belief that myomectomy is important. He or she should be skilled in the technique, and know microsurgical techniques for preventing adhesions.

.   .   .

Overall Complications. While multiple myomectomy is undoubtedly more difficult for the surgeon, is it really worse on the patient? Bonney's series showed a mortality rate similar to that for hysterectomy. Since myomectomy has been so out of favor in the United States, we must look to other countries to find enough myomectomies to get a clear idea of the complication rate.

In Trinidad, for example, the rate of complications in 1966 was virtually the same in 100 patients who underwent myomectomy and 100 who underwent hysterectomy.[23] At Benin Teaching Hospital in Nigeria no patients of 122 who underwent myomectomy died, compared to 2 patients of 58 who had hysterectomies.[24] Complications, except for blood loss, were also more frequent in the hysterectomy group.

This doesn't necessarily mean that the immediate complications of myomectomy are less than those of hysterectomy, since in both cases the patients who underwent hysterectomy were somewhat older and therefore more likely to have problems. It does, however, cast doubt upon the widely held belief that myomectomy is the more dangerous operation. "Myomectomy is said to be more dangerous than hysterectomy," states a 1975 British gynecology textbook, "but this is not true for present-day surgery."[25]

CESAREAN SECTION AFTER MYOMECTOMY

When I first saw a gynecologist upon returning to the United States, she asked me if my uterine cavity had been entered during the myomectomy in France. The reason was that if it had, any children would probably need to be delivered by cesarean section.

I dutifully asked my French surgeon, and he replied that no, it hadn't, that the fibroids had simply been scraped off the outside. He told me then that French surgeons feel the uterus can withstand six such myomectomies without making a cesarean delivery necessary.

Most gynecologists would agree that if the uterine cavity has been entered, children should be delivered by cesarean. One study from Trinidad showed a 12.5 percent incidence of uterine rupture during pregnancy in patients who had had a myomectomy in which the uterine cavity had been entered.[26]

These authors advised that while some women with a uterine scar extending through the uterus could deliver vaginally without any problem, the risk of the scar coming apart is fairly great, and "the safest and most logical step would be an elective cesarean section at thirty-eight weeks gestations with careful monitoring from twenty-eight weeks onwards. This latter precaution is wise because all four instances of uterine rupture in our series occurred after twenty-eight weeks and before the onset of labour."

Even those who no longer believe in the rule "Once a cesarean, always a cesarean" point out that myomectomy scars are not the same as the scars from prior cesarean sections, since they may have to be made where the fibroids are, not at the place where healing will be strongest.

But again, this is not an absolute. Dr. Winston says, "In some cases where I have done both the surgery and am delivering the patient, and if she seems to be doing beautifully, I might take the chance of delivering vaginally." Dr. García points out that in many such women vaginal delivery could be attempted, as long as an emergency team was standing by.

Clearly, it's better to have to have a cesarean than not to be able to have a child at all, and the fact that children will have to be born by cesarean section should not be used as an argument to recommend hysterectomy over myomectomy, as it sometimes is.

HYSTEROSCOPIC MYOMECTOMY

A few gynecologists have learned a technique whereby fibroids inside the uterus, known as submucous fibroids, can be removed through the vagina in a procedure known as hysteroscopic myomectomy.[27]

Developed by Robert Neuwirth, M.D., head of obstetrics and gynecology at St. Luke's Hospital in New York City, the procedure doesn't require you to stay very long in the hospital or to have a cesarean if you later have a child. Nor does it leave an abdominal scar.

Dr. Neuwirth has performed well over 100 hysteroscopic myomectomies, he said, and in only two was it necessary to open the abdomen during the procedure.

Bleeding returned to normal in about 80 to 90 percent of the women, Dr. Neuwirth reported, and about half of the younger women who were trying to become pregnant conceived.

In the older woman who doesn't want further pregnancies, Dr. Neuwirth said, the endometrium can be destroyed at the same time the myoma is removed (see chapter 5), abolishing menstruation without hysterectomy.

The main reason hysteroscopic myomectomy cannot be performed, he said, is a very large uterus.

When Leonore was in her mid-forties, she began to bleed heavily, so heavily that she was always worried about staining her clothes no matter how many pads and tampons she used. She also became anemic and weak, once fainting in her doctor's office. She had two D & Cs in an attempt to correct the bleeding. She was prepared to undergo a hysterectomy, feeling there was no other choice, but it was postponed when she developed a viral infection.

In the meantime a relative heard Dr. Neuwirth on television and told Leonore. She saw Dr. Neuwirth, who examined her in his office by inserting the hysteroscope, a lighted tube that allowed him to see into her uterus. While the procedure was uncomfortable, it was not really painful because she had been given a local anesthetic.

Dr. Neuwirth determined that Leonore did indeed have a submucous fibroid, and she entered the hospital for another hysteroscopy, this time to remove the fibroid. This procedure was performed under general anesthesia, and Dr. Neuwirth at the same time cauterized the endometrium. Leonore was in the hospital about two days and had no side effects, nor did she need to recuperate when she got out of the hospital. Two years later she developed bleeding again, and another fibroid was removed in the same way. Leonore is now fifty-eight, and has had no further problems and has not needed a hysterectomy.

DRUG TREATMENTS FOR FIBROIDS

Most gynecologists say there is no drug treatment for fibroids. Some, such as Dr. Hutchins, say they sometimes have good luck using large doses of progestagens. In theory this should work; it does in animals. In humans, the data are less clear.[28] In any case, progestagens can help treat the bleeding disorders often associated with fibroids (see chapter 5), so you might discuss with your doctor trying it for a while if you have heavy bleeding due to fibroids and aren't ready for surgery.

Progestagens can, however, alter fibroids in a way that makes them look cancerous when they really aren't: if you take progestagens and *then* have surgery, you could get a false diagnosis of cancer.[29]

Recently, however, several centers in the United States and around the world have been experimenting with GnRH analogs.[30] There seems to be no doubt that in many cases, giving women these drugs dramatically shrinks their fibroids by producing a reversible menopause. Dr. Rodolphe Maheux of the Center for Endocrinology of Reproduction and Infertility of the Saint-François d'Assise Hospital in Quebec, reported in 1985 that of twelve fibroids in ten women treated with subcutaneous injections three times daily for one week and then daily for the six-month treatment period, seven of the fibroids showed a marked regression in size, two shrank to the point where they could no longer be detected, and the volume of the other five diminished by an average of 80 percent.[31]

Dr. Maheux has now used GnRH analogs on about forty patients with good results. But not all fibroids respond. Most grow back in size after the drug has been discontinued, and the drug cannot be given indefinitely because the artificial menopause provoked will cause such menopausal symptoms as bone loss. In addition, it is expensive and difficult to take, although a nasal spray is being developed. So far, these problems make the drug impractical in most patients.

There are, however, Dr. Maheux pointed out, two types of patients who might benefit. One is the woman of about forty-five, who has just a few more years to go until menopause, and the other is the young woman with large fibroids scheduled for myomectomy.

"We know that the surgical prognostic of myomectomy is directly affected by the volume of the tumor," he said. If you have a big fibroid, "you don't have a good prognosis for post-myomectomy fertility." If the tumor can be shrunk prior to my-omectomy by GnRH analogs, the chances of future conception may be better.

The tumors may even shrink to the size where they can be removed through the laparoscope, a tube that is inserted through tiny incisions in the abdomen, he said, avoiding major surgery altogether.

GnRH analogs are available in this country, but the Food and Drug Administration has approved them only for the treatment of prostate cancer. Once a drug is on the market, however, doctors can prescribe it for any disease they want to, although they should tell you that the drug is being used experimentally.[32] Some universities are currently researching this drug, and if you think you might be a good candidate for such experimental treatment, you might contact the department of obstetrics and gynecology at your local medical school.

Dr. Schinfeld, who occasionally uses GnRH analogs, explained some of the pros and cons: "There are risks from the drug, for example, osteoporosis, hot flashes, and vaginal dryness. It's a good drug, but like any drug you find out that many women can't take it or tolerate it. It should really be used at this moment for from four to six months." While the drug currently must be given by subcutaneous injection and costs about $134 per week, Dr. Schinfeld hopes the newer nasal spray will be less expensive. "But I would still think it would be $60 to $80 a month minimum."

Summing Up

If you have fibroids, you are not alone: from 30 to 50 percent of all women have them, although they may not be aware of them.

If your fibroids are small and not causing symptoms, you need no treatment whatsoever, although your gynecologist may wish to have you come in slightly more often in order to keep an eye on their size.

If your fibroids make your uterus as large as it would be if you were three months pregnant, or if they are causing symptoms such as pain, bleeding, urinary obstruction, or infertility, you may want them treated.

Your doctor may tell you that hysterectomy is the only treatment, but the fibroids can almost always be removed in an operation known as myomectomy. If myomectomy is done by someone skilled in the technique, it should cause no more complications than hysterectomy, and you will still have your uterus.

If fibroids inside your uterus are causing you to bleed heavily, you might want to consider a lesser surgical procedure known as hysteroscopic myomectomy.

An experimental drug known as GnRH analog has been shown to shrink fibroids dramatically. While this drug is expensive and has a number of complications, it may become more widely used in the future.

Chapter 5

Heavy Bleeding—
Regular or Not

"I had stained so many easy chairs, straight-back chairs, sofas, couches, carpets, beds! I had left behind me so many puddles, spots, spotlets, splashes and droplets, in so many living rooms, dining rooms, anterooms, halls, swimming pools, buses, and other places. I could no longer go out." Marie Cardinal, The Words to Say It (1983)

When Anne, a financial journalist, found her periods becoming heavier and more painful as she reached her forties, she first thought, in the tradition of her New England background, that she should be stoic and "tough it out." She then decided to bring up the problem with her gynecologist, a woman about Anne's age, in case it was a sign that something was wrong. Perhaps, she thought, she could get some medication that might help.

"I can still remember very vividly what she said to me," Anne recalled. "She said, 'Well, you should consider yourself lucky, there are people who suffer even more than you, whose periods are longer and worse.' The inference for me was, 'Don't complain.' Then she said, 'There's always the option of having a hysterectomy.'

"I don't know why," said Anne, "but it just hit me like cold, cold weather. . . . I thought, 'Help! That's the last thing I'm going to consider.' I'm not afraid of having this kind of operation if it makes sense, but her suggestion just seemed gratuitous."

Anne decided to talk to her friends. One said that her gynecologist had given her a D & C [dilatation and curettage, a scraping of the inner lining of the uterus] that had helped. Interestingly enough, the gynecologist had also encouraged her to meditate, and Anne's friend had learned Transcendental Meditation, which did in fact help. "There's a whole stress-related element to bleeding," said Anne, who noticed that when she herself was under stress her bleeding got worse. Depression also makes her periods worse, and Anne notes that depression is one of the ways she experiences stress.

Anne changed gynecologists. Her new one prescribed one multivitamin pill a day and a type of iron pill that is well absorbed from the intestine to help counteract the anemia that was resulting from the heavy bleeding. He also told Anne to take vitamin K when the bleeding was heavy and gave her a chart to mark down the heavy days of her period. "I think there's something psychologically valid about keeping track," Anne said. "This little card has made a difference. I'm much more conscious of what's going on."

While her periods are still somewhat heavy and painful, they seem to be better, and her new doctor has reassured her that they will try other diagnostic methods and treatments before considering a hysterectomy.

Heavy or irregular menstrual bleeding is the second most frequent cause of hysterectomy in the United States, probably because gynecologists like Anne's first one don't look for other solutions. There are no magical ones that work perfectly for everyone, but there are a variety of ways to treat heavy bleeding ranging from vitamin and iron therapy to destruction of the lining of the uterus by either cautery or laser. "Hysterectomy is rarely indicated," wrote Jamil A. Fayez, M.D., chief of reproductive endocrinology at Bowman Gray School of Medicine in Winston-Salem, North Carolina. It is the last resort for the treatment of abnormal bleeding in women around the menopause, and "is indicated only when all other methods fail."[1]

THE MENSTRUAL CYCLE

To understand abnormal bleeding, one must understand the normal menstrual cycle, which is so wonderfully complex that scientists still don't quite understand how it works. Try to bear with me as I explain what is known about both normal and abnormal periods: this information can help explain why certain treatments may or may not work for you.

The normal menstrual cycle consists of three phases. Starting shortly after menstruation itself is the *proliferative* phase, sometimes called the *follicular* phase. During this phase, the pituitary gland directs the ovary to mature one of its egg follicles. It also directs the ovary to produce estrogen, which causes the inner lining of the uterus, the endometrium, to grow or proliferate. Estrogen directs the growth of small arteries that bring blood to the uterus, and it causes these arteries to dilate.

At about the fourteenth day after the beginning of menstruation the pituitary sends a signal to the ovary to release an egg, a process known as ovulation. The empty space that results in the ovary when the egg is released fills with a yellow substance and is known as a corpus luteum (yellow body). The ovary continues to secrete estrogen, but the corpus luteum produces progesterone in addition, which has several important effects on the lining of the uterus. It is to some extent an anti-estrogen, so it prevents the lining of the uterus from growing any larger. It also directs the lining to begin secreting glycogen, which in the case of pregnancy would nourish the growing fetus. Because progesterone directs the lining to secrete, this phase is often referred to as the *secretory* phase, or if you are more concerned about what is happening in the ovary, the *luteal* phase. Progesterone also causes the small arteries to constrict.

If fertilization occurs, the ovary will continue to secrete estrogen and progesterone. If fertilization does not occur, this message will reach the pituitary about fourteen days later. The pituitary directs the ovary to stop producing hormones, since they are not needed for pregnancy. It is this sudden withdrawal of both estrogen and progesterone that results in menstruation one or two days later.

The withdrawal of the hormones makes it impossible for the lining of the uterus, which has by now grown from about half a millimeter to about five millimeters thick, to survive. As it begins to break down, the small arteries are also broken and bleed, the process we know as menstruation.

While the thickening lining of the endometrium has been sequestered in the uterus for several weeks, the blood has not; the blood that is shed during menstruation was just a few minutes before circulating throughout the body.

The amount of blood you lose, therefore, depends both on the hormonal stimulation that has taken place throughout the previous month *and* on what happens to your body at the moment of menstruation.

Bleeding from the endometrium is somewhat different from bleeding from a cut finger. It used to be thought that menstrual blood didn't clot at all, but now it appears that it does clot, but in a slightly different, less complete way. When a finger bleeds, platelets and fibrin cause the formation of a blood clot that totally covers the wound and prevents further bleeding. But the uterus bleeds in layers, and while platelets and fibrin are deposited, they do not completely seal off the bleeding but form a little plug that the blood can leak around. A little later, another layer of the endometrium breaks off and more platelet and fibrin are deposited.[2] "It's almost like having an open wound that heals and then starts bleeding again," said Laurence Demers, M.D., a professor of pathology at Hershey Medical Center in Hershey, Pennsylvania. This process continues, a layer at a time, until all the lining is shed. With the stimulation of estrogen, the whole process starts again.

HEAVY BUT REGULAR BLEEDING

Abnormalities of menstruation that may lead to hysterectomy are either heavy bleeding during periods that are otherwise regular, known as *menorrhagia*, or bleeding that is irregular and often heavy, known as *dysfunctional uterine bleeding*.

Heavy, regular periods are not usually dangerous: they are more of a bother than anything else. While you should report them to your gynecologist, and he or she may want to perform further diagnostic tests, heavy periods are rarely a sign of cancer or indeed anything else very serious. The exception may be in young girls who have just started menstruating: here, heavy periods may be the first sign that their blood is unable to coagulate normally.[3] A diagnostic D & C may or may not be recommended, depending on a variety of other factors. In general, a D & C is not recommended in women under the age of thirty-five, since it can lead to scarring of the uterus that could interfere with childbearing. More diagnostic tests may be indicated for the older woman, who runs a greater risk of cancer.

Sometimes heavy periods are caused by fibroid tumors inside the uterus, which (as we saw in chapter 4) can be treated by myomectomy, sometimes done through a hysteroscope. In other cases, the bleeding may be due to more stimulation by estrogen than by progesterone. But in many cases doctors don't have a clue as to why some women start having very heavy periods.

"There's no question but that heavy bleeding can occur when the ovulation is normal and the luteal phase is normal," said Gerald F. Joseph, Jr., M.D., associate chairman of obstetrics and gynecology at the Ochsner Clinic in New Orleans. "It's a different kind of bleeding. We see a good percentage of women who have had lots of babies, especially in their middle to later thirties, who complain of cyclic, regular menstrual periods that are just very, very heavy, heavier than anything they have been accustomed to."

When should bleeding be considered heavy? Researchers define heavy bleeding as losing more than eighty milliliters of menstrual fluid (about one-third of a cup) each menstrual period.[4] Most of us, of course, do not measure our menstrual flow, and many doctors feel that the number of tampons and sanitary napkins we use tells more about our fastidiousness than about how heavy our flow is. Many also feel that our estimation of whether our flow is light or heavy is unreliable. But Paula Pendergrass, M.D., who did several studies on menstrual flow when she was an associate professor of anatomy at Wright State University Medical School in Dayton, Ohio, looked at whether a woman considered her flow light, medium, or heavy and then actually measured the flow. "There wasn't any correlation between the people who said they were light or moderate. But the people who said they were heavy—they were heavy. If a woman tells you she has heavy flow, then the chances are good that she does indeed."

In general, said Dr. Joseph, there's no reason that heavy bleeding needs to be treated unless you become anemic. You do, of course, run the risk of staining your clothes, and many women report avoiding slacks, particularly light-colored ones, or indeed anything other than dark skirts during their periods. What you may not realize is that some gynecologists believe that restricting your wardrobe in this fashion can be so handicapping to a woman that it justifies hysterectomy.

One southern gynecologist, for example, told me: "Since I live in the South, I have girls who tell me in the summer they're afraid of wearing white dresses because they bleed through them and that's socially handicapping. And if that's a real bother to them, then I think doctors need to be concerned in trying to fix it whatever way they can."

Do white dresses explain the fact that the southern states have the highest hysterectomy rate in the country? And do women who have hysterectomies for this reason fully understand that their inability to wear white dresses on certain days is their only serious problem? If they do, and decide on a hysterectomy being fully informed of the risks, I have no objection. What concerns me more is that many women duly report any staining as a measure of how heavily they are bleeding when their real concern is that something is wrong, perhaps cancer. Blood draws upon strong emotions that we often cannot deal with in a totally rational manner, and while the physician may believe a woman wants a hysterectomy in order to wear white dresses, the woman may in fact be afraid of cancer and it may not occur to her that a gynecologist could recommend major surgery for such a frivolous reason. I have often dutifully reported a symptom to a physician not because the symptom was bothering me particularly but because I though it might be useful in making a diagnosis. The physician's response has often been to assume that I want treatment for the symptom and to write out a prescription.

Marilyn, a public relations director of a large Canadian concern, had a hysterectomy at age forty for fibroids, five years after her myomectomy. She was pleased with the hysterectomy, thought she should have skipped the myomectomy and had the hysterectomy five years earlier, and was relieved to not have to worry about becoming pregnant.

At her postoperative visit her gynecologist, a young woman, said, "Aren't you happy to be able to wear anything you want now?"

"I was shocked," said Marilyn, "that she could consider this important enough to even talk about. That wasn't *why I had the operation."*

ANEMIA

In general the only other problem you risk with heavy periods is anemia, or a relative lack of the oxygen-carrying substance hemoglobin in the blood.

Doctors don't seem to agree what constitutes anemia and when it should be treated. A blood hemoglobin that is moderately low may in fact protect against heart attack. Some think a hemoglobin of less than twelve grams per 100 milliliters should be treated by iron supplements, while others would say ten. At eight, most doctors would begin to get worried, according to Dr. Demers.

At eight grams per 100 milliliters you may well have symptoms of fatigue and rapid heart rate from the anemia. In addition, should you be injured in an accident or have surgery, your reserves would be even further depleted.

One reason to seriously consider taking iron supplements if you have heavy periods is that there is evidence that the iron pills may not only correct the anemia but also actually make your periods lighter.

In 1964, Melvin L. Taymor, M.D., and his colleagues published a study in which half the patients were given iron pills and half a placebo, with neither patients nor their doctors knowing which was which.[5] Three-quarters of patients treated with iron reported less bleeding, compared to about one-third treated with the placebo. Most of the patients in whom the iron didn't work had something else wrong with them, such as fibroids.

"Iron deficiency from whatever cause may lead to menorrhagia, and menorrhagia in turn produces a more severe iron deficiency," Dr. Taymor concluded. "Therapy with iron breaks this vicious cycle."

Since the study was published in 1964, and very few of the gynecologists I talked to seemed to know about it, I telephoned Dr. Taymor, now chief of the division of reproductive endocrinology at Beth Israel Hospital in Boston, to see why. Perhaps in the interim another study had shown his results incorrect? Dr. Taymor said that as far as he knew they were still valid, just not widely known. Should a woman with heavy periods treat herself with iron? Dr. Taymor's response was that it certainly can't hurt to do so and that it may in fact help. Iron plays a number of roles in the body besides carrying oxygen in the blood, and it may in some way help the uterine muscles to contract, he suggested, turning off the bleeding once it has started. One British paper I came upon suggested that although taking iron when you aren't menstruating helps decrease the flow, taking it *during* your period may make it heavier.[6]

There is also some evidence that vitamin A deficiency may lead to heavy bleeding. The chief proponent of this view is Dr. D. M. Lithgow of South Africa, who published a study several years ago in the *South African Medical Journal* claiming that large doses of vitamin A could cure heavy bleeding.[7] It should be noted here that Dr. Lithgow believes that South African whites have a high rate of such deficiency because of the large amount of sunshine they receive. However, he believes that vitamin A should help if you are deficient for whatever reason, which can be because you don't ingest enough of it, have had a recent infection, consume alcohol excessively, or have certain intestinal diseases. Signs of vitamin A deficiency are nail shadowing, furred tongue, dry cervix, dry, lusterless hair, and black rings around the eyes.

While Dr. Lithgow used large doses—25,000 international units—to treat his patients with heavy bleeding, this treatment may not be without dangers, particularly as there is evidence that vitamin A may cause birth defects.[8] In addition, too much carotene, the compound related to vitamin A that is found in green vegetables, can actually cause menstrual difficulties.[9] But if for some reason you are bleeding heavily and feel you might be deficient in vitamin A, it shouldn't hurt to make sure that you eat several servings of green or yellow vegetables a week. As we shall see in chapter 7, this may also help keep your cervix healthy.

Sometimes medication taken for other conditions can cause your periods to become heavier. Nifedipine, for example, which is prescribed for high blood pressure, for Raynaud's syndrome, and sometimes for menstrual cramps, has sometimes been found to make the periods heavier.[10] Patients put on anticoagulant medication such as coumadin or heparin to prevent heart attacks or strokes might also have heavier periods.[11] If you take prescription drugs, be sure to discuss with your physician whether one of them might be causing your heavy periods. And if you take nonprescription drugs frequently, you might keep a log to see if there's any correlation between what you take and the heaviness of your periods.

TREATMENT OPTIONS

You may, of course, wish to stick to iron pills, and unless you are severely anemic there's really no reason that you need to take anything else. But here are treatments that have been found to reduce the amount of menstrual bleeding for some women.

·   ·   ·

Antiprostaglandins. These are the drugs that for many of us have abolished menstrual cramps. But while their role in lessening the pain of menstruation has been fairly well established, their ability to reduce the amount of bleeding itself has been more controversial. Some reports have even indicated that they might make the bleeding irregular, particularly if taken a few days before the period starts.[12]

A very recent report from Scandinavia sheds some light on why the effect of these drugs on bleeding has been hard to determine.[13] This report looked at the effect of the drugs on women with and without fibroids who were bleeding heavily. In the women with fibroids, the antiprostaglandins had no effect. But in the women without fibroids, the drug reduced the bleeding by 36 percent when taken for five days starting on the first day of the period. These drugs are available in this country (Anaprox is a common one), and some of them are even available without a prescription (Advil).

Antihistamines. A more offbeat method that you might want to try is over-the-counter antihistamines. Dr. Pendergrass and her co-workers studied the effect of antihistamines and found that they dramatically reduced menstrual blood loss in some women.[14] Histamines are chemicals that cause congestion, and they tend to rise when estrogen levels fall, explaining why asthma sufferers often have increased discomfort just before their periods. Dr. Pendergrass explained that histamines have also been found in animal studies to cause congestion of the blood vessels in the uterus and to contract the uterine muscle. Both actions could theoretically increase menstrual flow, and blocking these actions with antihistamines should be able to decrease it, she said.

To test how histamine worked in women, Dr. Pendergrass and her co-workers studied fifty women aged eighteen to forty-four in whom the amount of menstrual loss was measured for two periods. The women were then divided into two groups to receive either an antihistamine (in this case, chlorpheniramine maleate, or Teldrin) or a placebo. Subjects were instructed to take the first capsule when the first spots of their period began and to take another capsule every twelve hours for three days, a total of six capsules.

When the results were analyzed, they showed that although antihistamines had reduced menstrual flow in the group as a whole, the results were not statistically significant, meaning that they could have occurred by chance. Dr. Pendergrass noted that in such a small sample it is difficult to attain statistical significance.

What is more interesting, however, is that a few individuals reacted dramatically, decreasing their menstrual flow by as much as 70 percent. Fifteen subjects decreased their flow, an average of 35 percent, which was twice as much as in the group receiving a placebo.

Such individual responses seem to be characteristic of responses to antihistamines in general, Dr. Pendergrass noted.

Would it be dangerous for a woman who has heavy bleeding with no evidence of anything else wrong to try treating herself with antihistamines? Dr. Pendergrass thought not. "If they don't make you drowsy and you don't lose work, then yes, I would say try it," she said. A number of good antihistamines can be purchased over the counter, some of which are now reported not to cause drowsiness, and they would probably need to be taken only for the first day or two of the period.

Hormonal Treatments. If you have ever taken birth-control pills, you know they dramatically reduce the amount of blood lost during each period. Since they are not generally recommended for women over the age of thirty-five or forty, this limits their use since it is at this age that periods most often become heavy.

Progestagens such as Provera are sometimes used in older women, particularly in those with irregular bleeding, as we shall see later. But since progestagens are one component of the birth-control pill, it's not clear that they are any safer. Some physicians are willing to consider using birth-control pills in older women, particularly if they are nonsmokers.

Danazol is another possible remedy. A derivative of testosterone, it is most commonly used in endometriosis; its troublesome side effects will be discussed in chapter 11. Endometriosis patients typically receive 800 milligrams a day, but English researchers have found that doses as low as 100 milligrams can be used to control bleeding.[15] These researchers found that side effects were troublesome only in those receiving doses of 400 milligrams or more. "The only side effects noted by women on 200 milligrams were mild acne and mild decrease in breast size," they wrote. Danazol will produce birth defects if taken during pregnancy, however, and the effect on bleeding will disappear once the drug is discontinued. It's best used by women who have really heavy bleeding and haven't found anything else that works.

GnRH analogs (see the description of their action on page 181) also seem to be quite effective in reducing blood loss in ovulating women, but again, the effect is lost once the drug is stopped. One study showed it reduced menstrual losses of 95 to 198 milliliters per month to between 4 and 30 milliliters.[16] In one pilot study where the drug was given via nasal spray, the most serious side effect was nasal irritation. At this point, though, GnRH analogs are very, very expensive and must be considered experimental.

Promising Developments. Two drugs widely used in Europe for the treatment of heavy bleeding, ethamsylate and tranexamic acid, may soon be on the market here.

Tranexamic acid is used routinely in Sweden and many other countries, according to Dr. Lennart Nilsson, a retired professor of gynecology at the University of Gothenburg, Sweden. It works by stabilizing the clotting mechanism within the uterus. In one trial led by Dr. Nilsson, it reduced the menstrual blood loss by 50 percent.[17] According to the drug company that makes it, it is expected to be registered in the United States soon, although heavy bleeding will not be given as an official reason to prescribe the drug. If you are bleeding severely enough to be considering hysterectomy, however, you might ask your doctor about it, since once a drug is approved for one indication it can be prescribed for others.

Ethamsylate works by increasing the resistance of the capillaries so that they don't allow so much blood to escape. Just before the menstrual cycle and in the first two or three days of it, the blood vessels in the uterus begin to break down and become more fragile due to the sudden withdrawal of estrogen. In one British trial, ethamsylate reduced the mean menstrual blood loss by 50 percent in patients with primary menorrhagia, and by 19 percent in patients using an IUD.[18] Only one of the twenty-six patients reported any side effects at all. According to literature supplied to me by the drug company that markets ethamsylate in the United Kingdom under the trade name Dicynene, there are no known reasons why a woman could not use the drug, and it is well tolerated even in high dosage or during prolonged treatment. It is not, however, marketed in the United States, although the manufacturer, Delandale Laboratories, is considering applying to the FDA.

IRREGULAR BLEEDING

Janet had always had heavy periods, but as long as they were regular she found she could manage. She had her first child at the age of forty, and about two years later her periods became extremely heavy. After two years, "my schedule started to get screwy too. I might have an episode of heavy bleeding three weeks after the previous one or six weeks after it."

Janet consulted a gynecologist, who felt some fibroids in her uterus and thought the heavy bleeding was probably due both to these and to the fact that Janet was nearing menopause. Eventually she developed anemia and became very weak. "One day I became terrified at how weak I felt. I called the gynecologist and she immediately put me in the hospital for a D & C. My blood count was so low I had to have three pints of blood."

While the gynecologist suggested that Janet seriously consider a hysterectomy, she didn't press her, and made it clear that the only issue was really how uncomfortable Janet herself was. Because she was very busy at work at the time, Janet scheduled a hysterectomy for a few months later. While the gynecologist didn't believe that progestagen would work, she nevertheless prescribed it. "Coincidentally or not, my schedules did adjust," Janet said. "Suddenly I was on a regular schedule, and because I was treating the anemia I was much stronger. The bleeding was still very heavy, but being able to predict my periods made a big difference." She canceled the hysterectomy, but began bleeding again after about six months. While she considered having a procedure known as laser ablation of the endometrium, in which the inner lining of the uterus is destroyed, she eventually rejected it because her gynecologist felt that as a new procedure some of the problems hadn't yet been ironed out. She finally decided on a vaginal hysterectomy, which went well. She felt she had explored her options, given alternatives a try, and that vaginal hysterectomy was really the best solution for her.

DYSFUNCTIONAL UTERINE BLEEDING

Janet's change from heavy, regular periods to irregular periods made a dramatic difference in her life. But irregularity is more than just an added nuisance; it usually requires a higher degree of medical attention. Rarely does it indicate cancer. More commonly it indicates that you are not ovulating, which, over time, may lead to precancerous changes of the endometrium or even cancer itself.

If you don't ovulate, you can't become pregnant, but in addition the whole delicate balance of estrogen and progesterone is upset. The continuous stimulation of the endometrium by estrogen without the moderating effects of progesterone causes it to continue to grow. Finally, either because it outgrows its blood supply or the estrogen level suddenly drops, the lining of the uterus is shed in an uncontrolled manner, leading to heavy bleeding.

Ovulation is a very delicate process that can be stopped by a variety of factors. Many physical illnesses will block it, as will being too fat or too thin, or exercising too much. Stress can also interfere with ovulation by raising the level of certain chemicals in the body.[19]

Dysfunctional bleeding is also a common symptom of endometriosis, probably because the endometrial implants on the ovary interfere with hormone production.

For many years, Monique, a biochemist, had low-grade fever and was exhausted most of the time. "You know how you feel when you have the flu? That's how I felt." When she was thirty-three, Monique began to have dysfunctional bleeding, which the gynecologist told her was typical for a woman her age. He started a D & C but perforated her uterus and didn't complete the procedure, a fact, incidentally, of which Monique was unaware until another gynecologist got the report and told her. When she was thirty-eight, she learned she had endometriosis and eventually was treated by videolaserlaparoscopy, which eliminated many of her symptoms (see chapter 11).

Even without physical or mental stress, anovulatory cycles —or cycles during which ovulation does not occur—are common at both ends of the reproductive years: in teenagers just starting their periods and in women nearing menopause. While 90 percent of women will have regular periods up to the age of forty, only 10 percent will remain regular up to menopause.[20] Some gynecologists refer to these years of irregular bleeding as the premenopause.

If you bleed irregularly and aren't ovulating, your doctor will probably want to treat you, either by reestablishing ovulation so the body can make its own progesterone or by replacing the progesterone.

Reestablishing ovulation can be done either by dealing with underlying physical disease, reducing emotional stress, or giving a fertility drug such as clomiphene citrate. Clomiphene has been found to cause fibroid tumors to grow rapidly, though, so it should be used with caution if you have fibroids.[21]

For women on the verge of menopause, the most common treatment is the administration of synthetic forms of progesterone known as progestins or progestagens. Progestagens will often work quite well for a while, often long enough to carry you through to menopause. Unfortunately, as we saw in chapter 2, they can make you depressed. Also unfortunately, they may only work for several months before the bleeding starts again, as in Janet's case. "It's like using diuretics," said Dr. García. "Your kidneys compensate after a while, and you have to keep increasing the dosage."

But many women will find these few months long enough to carry them through.

Your doctor may also suggest birth-control pills, since while they block ovulation, they do provide both estrogen and progesterone stimulation to the uterus. Birth-control pills are associated with an increased risk of stroke and heart attack in older women and smokers, but it's simply not known whether they are worse than progestagens.

A smaller group of women experience dysfunctional uterine bleeding even though they are ovulating. In these women, the amount of progesterone produced is considered inadequate to sufficiently counteract the effects of estrogen, and progesterone may be prescribed.

WILL A D & C HELP?

Dilatation and curettage, as I've said, is sometimes used in dysfunctional bleeding as a diagnostic method to rule out cancer. In certain cases, the D & C is also therapeutic and helps the bleeding. But the gynecologists I surveyed believe that as therapy D & Cs are pretty much hit or miss. Unless a small submucous fibroid or polyp has been causing the bleeding and it is removed during the D & C, all the procedure does is reduce bleeding for about one cycle. After that bleeding will return to what it was before or become even heavier for a cycle or two. Nevertheless, many gynecologists would consider it worth trying a few times if medical treatment doesn't work.

If nothing else has worked, there is still one alternative to

hysterectomy for the woman who wants to stop bleeding heavily
—and who doesn't want children.

LASER ABLATION OF THE ENDOMETRIUM

Milton Goldrath, M.D., chairman of the department of obstetrics
and gynecology at Sinai Hospital of Detroit, Michigan, has pi-
oneered a technique known as laser ablation of the endometrium. In this technique, a YAG (yttrium, aluminum, and garnet)
laser, different from the carbon-dioxide laser used more commonly in gynecology, is used to destroy the endometrium, thus
ending menstrual bleeding once and for all.[22] At the 1986 meeting
of the American College of Obstetricians and Gynecologists, Dr.
Goldrath reported over 300 cases of laser ablation, 260 having at
least six months follow-up. These women were all candidates for
hysterectomy before their treatment based on the criteria of his
hospital, which he characterizes as strict. So far, only 10 women
who have undergone laser ablation have needed a hysterectomy,
he reported, about half of them because they were found to have
a condition related to endometriosis known as adenomyosis, in
which the inner lining of the uterus invades the other layers,
making it tender. About 97 percent of the results were considered
excellent, with some spotting a few days a month or no bleeding
at all.

The major advantage of this procedure is that it involves no
incision so it is not really surgery at all. "If you can do this as an
outpatient procedure you're saving the patient a lot of pain, disability, and loss of income," said Dr. Goldrath. In Detroit at least,
it costs about $5,000 to $6,000 less than a hysterectomy, he said,
although insurance companies may be less willing to pay because
they consider it an experimental procedure.

The YAG laser has recently been approved by the Food and
Drug Administration, and according to Dr. Daniell, there are
probably fifteen to twenty gynecologists around the country who
perform the procedure. Some gynecologists, such as Dr. Neuwirth, perform a similar procedure with cautery.

One possible complication that can occur with laser ablation is fluid overload, since fluid must be used and it may enter the bloodstream. In most cases this will simply mean an increased need to urinate for a while, but Dr. Goldrath reported two cases of pulmonary edema (water accumulation in the lungs) "which is a very frightening situation." In both cases, it was corrected with no untoward results. It's important to make sure that the anesthesiologist is skillful in dealing with this complication.

Another theoretical disadvantage of the procedure is that cancer could develop in the small amount of endometrium that is left, and detection would be difficult because the scar tissue would make it difficult to perform the endometrial biopsies that are used to check for this cancer.

Yet the theoretical risk of not being able to detect endometrial cancer must be put in perspective. The risk of developing endometrial cancer is 1 per 1,000 women per year, Dr. Goldrath points out, and laser ablation will certainly not increase that risk. In fact, it should decrease the risk significantly, since practically no endometrium is left after the procedure. Laser ablation should not be performed in women with precancerous changes in the uterus, however.

BLEEDING AFTER THE MENOPAUSE

If you begin bleeding after you have undergone menopause, you should definitely see your doctor, as such bleeding can be a sign of cancer. Keep in mind, though, that many doctors were taught —erroneously—that 50 percent of postmenopausal bleeding is due to cancer. Some therefore recommend hysterectomy without checking to see whether cancer has developed, even though more recent studies have shown that only about 7 percent of women who bleed after menopause have the disease.[23] So most cases of postmenopausal bleeding will not mean you have to have a hysterectomy.[24]

Summing Up

A common cause of hysterectomy is either heavy, regular bleeding or irregular bleeding. Heavy, regular bleeding is mostly a bother, although it can indicate the presence of fibroid tumors within the uterus and can lead to anemia. There are a variety of treatments for heavy bleeding, such as iron pills, antiprostaglandins, antihistamines, and hormones, which may or may not work for you.

Irregular bleeding is both more bothersome and potentially more dangerous. Since it nearly always results from a failure to ovulate, treatments are directed at either reestablishing ovulation, or replacing the progesterone that would normally be present following ovulation so that the estrogen in the body does not go unopposed.

If drug treatments fail and you do not wish to have more children, destruction of the inner lining of the uterus by laser is a new treatment that may help you avoid hysterectomy.

If you bleed after menopause, you should see your gynecologist, since this could be a sign of cancer. However, only about 7 percent of cases actually turn out to be cancer, so you will not necessarily have to have a hysterectomy even then.

Chapter 6

Hyperplasia
and Endometrial Cancer

"The primary reason that women are consenting to hysterectomy and oophorectomy is fear of cancer." Nora Coffey, president and founder, Hysterectomy Educational Resources and Services Foundation (HERS)

Debora, a food consultant and chef in her late thirties, was wearing white slacks the day she first hemorrhaged. The hemorrhages continued, often in public places such as delicatessens, taxicabs, or trains, and finally as her plane was landing in Rome, where she soaked not only the seat but the blankets brought by the stewardess. Her gynecologist, a woman, had originally told her not to worry, that such hemorrhaging was common at her age. Debora feels the gynecologist did not take good care of her, but she realizes that she may have minimized her symptoms when relating them to the doctor, partly because she feared the only treatment was hysterectomy. But after she started bleeding and hemorrhaging every day, she was eventually hospitalized and given three pints of blood and a diagnosis of adenomatous hyperplasia with atypia, a definitely precancerous condition. Her original doctor now told her she would have to have a hysterectomy plus radium therapy. The cancer specialist at Yale, where she was referred, didn't recommend radium, but he did recommend hysterectomy.

But Debora very badly wanted a child.

Remaining in contact with the cancer specialist at Yale, she started seeing a fertility specialist who put her on clomiphene citrate, a drug to induce ovulation, with the stipulation that she must have a D & C every three months to monitor the hyperplasia. After the second D & C, everyone was delighted. Debora's symptoms had cleared, and her hyperplasia improved considerably. She still expects to get D & Cs every three months but is quite willing to continue without the hysterectomy, at least for a while.

The same unopposed estrogen stimulation that leads to abnormal bleeding may, if left untreated, lead to a condition known as endometrial hyperplasia and, eventually, to endometrial cancer, a cancer that accounts for approximately 2 percent of all cancer deaths in women.[1] Because of the relationship of both hyperplasia and cancer to estrogen stimulation, many physicians consider hyperplasia a precancerous condition and will recommend hysterectomy for it. In addition, because hyperplasia is often diagnosed as carcinoma, many women who think they are having a hysterectomy for cancer really don't have cancer at all.

In fact:

- Only one type of hyperplasia, the type Debora had, seems to indicate a significantly increased risk of cancer.
- This type of hyperplasia can often be successfully treated with drugs, or by discontinuing estrogen-replacement therapy.
- If the drugs don't reverse the condition, some gynecologists consider close follow-up a reasonable option, though it does involve a calculated risk.

LANGUAGE PROBLEMS

"The classification of endometrial hyperplasia will get you into more trouble than anything else," J. Donald Woodruff, M.D., Richard W. Telinde Professor of Gynecologic Pathology at Johns

Hopkins University School of Medicine, told a session of the 1986 meeting of the American College of Obstetricians and Gynecologists. Why?

As Dr. Winston puts it, "One pathologist talking about endometrial hyperplasia and another pathologist listening to him have two different pictures in their mind." Barbara Chaitin, M.D., a pathologist at Montefiore Hospital in the Bronx, New York, confirmed this: "I was trained at Stanford, which tends to be conservative, and I would tend to label hyperplasia what others here might call carcinoma."

How you regard this variabilty of diagnosis might depend on whether you fear being undertreated more than you fear being overtreated. Certainly it might suggest that any diagnosis of either endometrial carcinoma or hyperplasia warrants a second opinion—preferably from a university or specialized cancer center.[2]

Dr. Woodruff, for example, pointed out that about one-third of the cases of diagnosed endometrial cancer are not cancer but hyperplasia. This partly accounts for the very good survival rates cited for endometrial cancer. "American Cancer Society figures show 2,300 deaths a year from endometrial cancer. There are 39,000 new cases a year. This gives a 93 percent five-year survival according to the American Cancer Society. The five-year survival is really more like 65 to 70 percent. About 10,000 to 15,000 of these cases are not cancer but are benign disease," he said.

THE ESTROGEN CONNECTION

Since hyperplasia and at least some types of endometrial cancer seem to be associated with an excess of unopposed estrogen, you will be at increased risk for both conditions if you have any condition that tends to increase estrogen or decrease progesterone. These include being overweight and a condition known as Stein-Leventhal syndrome, where the ovaries are cystic and do not ovulate.[3] Taking estrogens without progestagens at the menopause increases the risk, as did an earlier form of birth-control pills (now off the market) known as sequential pills.[4] Smoking decreases the risk by about half, probably because smoke reduces estrogen levels.[5] But before you take up smoking to prevent endometrial cancer keep in mind that smoking kills many more women through lung cancer and heart disease than it saves from endometrial cancer, and it increases your risk of cervical cancer as well!

It therefore follows that progestagen, which opposes the action of estrogen, can prevent and sometimes reverse hyperplasia.[6] Dr. David Gal and his co-workers at the University of Texas Health Science Center at Dallas found that they were able to reverse hyperplasias completely in 90 percent of the postmenopausal women they treated with a strong progestagen.[7] Some gynecologists report that they have even treated a few young women who have endometrial cancer with progestagen rather than hysterectomy.[8]

In fact, many hyperplasias don't need any treatment except close follow-up—they reverse spontaneously, sometimes following a diagnostic D & C. This is particularly true for types of hyperplasia not considered precancerous, known as simple or cystic hyperplasias.

Consider, for example, patients with simple hyperplasia treated by Robert J. Kurman, M.D., and his co-workers at the Armed Forces Institute of Pathology in Washington, D.C.[9] Eighty percent of the patients had a spontaneous regression following their diagnostic D & C and needed no further treatment. One of the ninety-three patients in this series did eventually develop cancer, but she did so eleven years and one pregnancy after her initial diagnosis of hyperplasia. She had a hysterectomy when the cancer was diagnosed, and was alive and free of disease twenty-eight years later.

If you, like Debora, have a diagnosis of atypical hyperplasia, or adenomatous hyperplasia with atypia, the chance is much greater that you will eventually develop an endometrial cancer. In Dr. Kurman's series, for example, about one-fourth of patients with this diagnosis eventually developed cancer. They had hysterectomies then, and none died of cancer. Other studies, however, have shown a higher risk of cancer with this type of hyperplasia.

If you are found to have adenomatous hyperplasia with atypia, you should accept that you have a precancerous condition that is best treated either by hysterectomy or by close follow-up that will mean fairly frequent sampling of the endometrium by a doctor who is competent to judge its condition. You may also be prescribed hormonal treatment. Endometrial biopsies can be taken either as a D & C, where hospitalization and anesthesia are usually required, or in a simpler office procedure. Some doctors give some type of painkiller for the office procedure and some don't: if you find it painful, don't hesitate to ask for something for the pain, either pills or a local anesthetic. You may decide you prefer a hysterectomy, but remember that that is your choice.

ENDOMETRIAL CANCER

If you do develop endometrial cancer and are sure of the diagnosis, hysterectomy would seem to be your best bet for survival. John Paul Micha, M.D., an assistant clinical professor of gynecological oncology at the UCLA Medical Center, who works at the Hoag Hospital Cancer Center in Newport Beach, California, points out that surgery gives a better cure rate than radiotherapy. Radiotherapy, he feels, is preferable only if you are a poor surgical risk, perhaps because of age or obesity. "But that's rare—very few patients today cannot make it through surgery with careful intensive-care monitoring. The only time I ever used radiation therapy instead of surgery was on a lady who weighed about 450 pounds and had had five heart attacks."

Since endometrial cancer is considered to be an estrogen-dependent cancer, your ovaries will be removed as well as your uterus and estrogen-replacement therapy will not usually be recommended. William Creasman, M.D., now chairman of the department of obstetrics and gynecology at the Medical University of South Carolina at Charleston, however, believes that patients treated for endometrial cancer can be given estrogen.[10] Of 221 patients with early endometrial cancer, 47 received estrogen after their cancer therapy and 174 did not. The group receiving estrogen in fact had a longer disease-free survival.

Dr. Creasman and his coauthors acknowledge that further studies are needed, but they note that there are really no data to support the widely held view that patients treated for endometrial cancer should not be given estrogen.

While endometrial carcinoma is by far the most common type of cancer of the body of the uterus, two others deserve mention. One is leiomyosarcoma, which occurs in about 1 of every 200,000 women per year and generally is not very curable.[11] It is usually diagnosed by a rapidly expanding uterine mass. The other is choriocarcinoma, in which a hysterectomy is practically never necessary any more.

A CANCER WHERE HYSTERECTOMY IS OBSOLETE

Choriocarcinoma is a rare tumor, the most serious phase of a group of conditions known as gestational trophoblastic disease in which pregnancy goes awry; rather than a baby, a tumor looking like a bunch of grapes develops. The first sympton is usually bleeding during pregnancy, with the blood having a prune-juice appearance. The uterus may also be larger or smaller than would normally be expected for the stage of pregnancy.

If left untreated, choriocarcinoma is a deadly tumor. But it is one cancer, unlike many others, where chemotherapy really works. It works so well, in fact, that instead of being given in addition to surgery, as most chemotherapy is, it is given instead of it: it's the chemotherapy that cures over 90 percent of choriocarcinoma patients, and removing the uterus is often not necessary, although a hysterectomy may reduce the amount of chemotherapy needed.[12]

In fact, removing the uterus actually may make more sense in an earlier phase of gestational trophoblastic disease known as invasive mole. Here, hysterectomy is an option because it will decrease the risk of eventually needing chemotherapy, probably from about 25 percent to 5 percent. "I think a lot of people in this situation would want the hysterectomy," said Dr. Micha. "They don't want to take the chance of having to take chemotherapyand potentially have all the adverse consequences of hair loss, infections, bleeding easily, and perhaps the risk of leukemia at a later time. There are certainly good arguments for doing hysterectomy in some of those patients if they've completed their family and they're informed of the situation. On the other hand, in a younger patient with no children, there's no need to do a hysterectomy unless they've failed chemotherapy. The prognosis would be no worse in the older patient; her priorities might simply be different."

Dr. Micha continued, "A lot of lay people don't realize how much cancer surgery, and how often cancer-related decisions, are not black and white—'You've got to have a hysterectomy, you've got to have radiation therapy.' " Instead, just as in other medical situations, it's a profit-and-loss situation where, with the right information, you may be able to increase your profits and minimize your losses.

Summing Up

If you get a diagnosis of endometrial hyperplasia, or cancer of the uterine lining, you may well want to get a second opinion from a pathologist who specializes in endometrial pathology, since there is a great deal of variation in diagnosis from one pathologist to another.

Only one type of hyperplasia, adenomatous hyperplasia, significantly increases your risk of cancer.

If you get a diagnosis of adenomatous hyperplasia with atypia, you may want to have a hysterectomy. However, in some cases this condition can be reversed with drug treatment. If you choose not to have a hysterectomy, you should have your endometrium sampled frequently to make certain the hyperplasia is not progressing to cancer.

If you have a definite cancer of the endometrium, hysterectomy will give you a better chance of surviving than radiotherapy.

If you have a rare form of uterine cancer known as choriocarcinoma, chemotherapy should be the treatment considered. Chemotherapy cures over 90 percent of these cancers, and you will not need a hysterectomy unless the chemotherapy does not work, although the operation might reduce the amount of chemotherapy needed.

Chapter 7

Cervical Changes, Including Cancer

"Regrettably, neither life nor the terminology of neoplasia is simple."
Stanley L. Robbins et al., *Basic Pathology* (1981)

Suppose your next Pap test comes back abnormal and you are told to see your gynecologist as soon as possible. Does this mean a hysterectomy will be necessary to save your life? In the vast majority of cases, the answer is an emphatic no. An abnormal Pap test shows precancerous and other changes of the cervix, that part of the uterus that lies in the upper part of the vagina. If left untreated these precancerous changes do mean that you run an increased risk of cervical cancer. But they can nearly always be treated much less radically than with a hysterectomy. Some cases of early cervical cancer can even be treated without hysterectomy. And if you have a real cervical cancer, you always have the option of radiotherapy, although, as we shall see, in frankly invasive cancer hysterectomy may be the better choice because it can spare the ovaries.

But you can dramatically reduce your risk of developing invasive cervical cancer by having regular Pap smears and by pursuing a variety of other measures.

WHAT'S IN A NAME?

Unfortunately, in the past, an abnormal Pap smear often did culminate in a hysterectomy, even though the Pap test usually picks up abnormalities years before they begin behaving like true cancers. This was particularly tragic since abnormal smears are not uncommon in women in their teens and twenties.[1]

The alarming-sounding terminology doctors have used in discussing changes of the cervix accounts for at least part of the problem. For years, the less significant-looking precancerous changes in the cervix have been referred to as dysplasia, and the more significant ones as carcinoma-in-situ. But there is no black-and-white dividing line between the two, and pathologists often say that one pathologist's dysplasia is another pathologist's carcinoma-in-situ.

The terminology, however, has sometimes led to distinctly different treatment for dysplasia and for carcinoma-in-situ. Dysplasia has sometimes not been treated at all. And the term carcinoma-in-situ has been sufficiently frightening to many doctors that they've recommended hysterectomy to patients frightened enough by the term to accept it. Actually the term is a contradiction: by definition carcinoma is invasive, that is, it invades neighboring cells and tissues and eventually takes them over. But by definition "in situ" means that invasion has not occurred, and the usual arsenal of treatments brought out to deal with cancer don't need to be used.

"Carcinoma-in-situ is a bad term because of its historical and clinical connotations," explained Ralph Richart, M.D., director of obstetrical and gynecological pathology at the Sloane Hospital for Women of Columbia Presbyterian Medical Center in New York City. "Clinicians for so many years took out those uteri. We need to break that pattern—and one of the ways to do it is with a terminology change."

As early as 1965 Dr. Richart proposed in an article that the terms be changed from "dysplasia" and "carcinoma-in-situ" to "cervical intra-epithelial neoplasia (CIN) grades I, II, and III."[2]

In part, the change was intended to show that the process of developing cervical cancer is a continuous one, with no distinct breaks between the stages. But it was also intended to prevent hysterectomies being performed on twenty-year-old women when they had a diagnosis of carcinoma-in-situ.

Has the new terminology worked? "The situation is changing," said Dr. Richart, "and in many places it has changed dramatically. We still find physicians who follow the old system: 'If it's dysplasia I don't have to do anything, if it's carcinoma-in-situ I'll take out her uterus.' There have been some substantial changes in the diagnosis and management of these lesions. But I don't think they're changed universally yet. And I think that's a shame."

TREATMENTS FOR CIN

In general, once the process of cervical changes that can lead to cancer has started, the progression is slow. Many of the precancerous lesions will revert to normal without any treatment at all, or with any type of manipulation of the cervix.[3] It's a bit like fixing a piece of machinery by kicking it—by rights this shouldn't work but sometimes it does. Small "punch" biopsies—removal of small amounts of tissue that could not possibly include all the abnormal cells—can provoke a return to normal, as can delivery of a child. Even taking Pap smears seemed to have a curative effect in one study, although Pap smears are done for the purpose of diagnosis, not cure.[4]

Lyudmila, a museum film curator, was thirty-three when she had her first abnormal Pap smear. Her doctor performed a colposcopy, a procedure in which the cervix is viewed through a magnifying instrument. He took biopsies, including some from her endocervical canal, the opening in the cervix that allows menstrual blood and babies to come out. The diagnosis that came back was mild dysplasia. The doctor recommended a cone biopsy, a minor surgical procedure in which a slice of the cervix is removed and studied for cancerous changes, although he

*indicated there was no particular hurry. Lyudmila sought a second opin-
ion, and eventually, after she read that heavy smokers like herself progress to cancer more rapidly, she went to a third doctor for the "cone."
The third doctor did not take his own biopsy but used the slides she
brought from the first doctor two years earlier.*

*Lyudmila had the "cone," and when the report came back, there
was absolutely nothing abnormal about her cervical tissue, which had
either regressed on its own or perhaps following the initial biopsy.*

*She is not sure she would really have needed the cone had the third
doctor taken his own biopsy, but found that with all three doctors she
was unable to get straight answers to her questions. She remains philo-
sophical, however: "That's the chance you take. You'd hate to get cervical
cancer a few years down the road."*

While precancerous changes can revert to normal on their
own, they cannot be counted on to do so, and untreated, they
definitely increase your risk of developing invasive cancer. One
physician, for example, found that patients with dysplasia had
1,600 times the normal risk of developing carcinoma-in-situ.[5] Of
patients with carcinoma-in-situ (or CIN III), one study showed
that 30 percent had developed invasive cancer by the tenth year
of follow-up and 80 percent had developed invasive cancer by
the thirtieth year of follow-up.[6]

As in the case of precancerous changes of the endometrium
(see chapter 6), precancerous changes can be followed and hysterectomy performed when invasive cancer does develop. But
most doctors would recommend that you treat the precancerous
changes rather than simply following them, since precancerous
cervical changes can be cured by fairly minor procedures such as
laser cauterization, cryosurgery (freezing), or sometimes cone biopsy. Most cases, in fact, can be treated in the doctor's office
with either freezing or the carbon-dioxide laser. Either method
works by destroying the abnormal cells, and both seem to be
about equally effective.[7]

I have never had either treatment, so I can't really vouch for
their painlessness. Most medical reports say that neither requires
painkillers or anesthesia. But when women in one English study

were asked whether they would have liked some form of pain relief during their laser treatment, many said they would have.[8] If you are scheduled for laser treatment, you might discuss the possibility of pain relief with your doctor. Indeed, if you want something for pain during any medical procedure, be sure to let your doctor know. Decisions as to what painkillers to use or whether to use painkillers at all are often made arbitrarily, with doctors deciding not on the basis of how much pain women feel but how much the doctors think they should feel. There is often a difference, and don't be shy about speaking up.

One laser or cryosurgery treatment will probably be enough to reverse the CIN: it is in about 85 to 90 percent of cases.[9] Occasionally, you may need a second treatment, and after two treatments 97 percent of patients are cured. If your Pap smear returns to normal and stays that way for a while, your risk of developing further cervical problems is only slightly higher than for the general population.[10] You will, of course, want to keep on having Pap smears at reasonable intervals, perhaps once a year.

Usually, these treatments are sufficient. A cone biopsy will be needed, however, if abnormal cells are found in the endocervical canal or if the results cannot be interpreted clearly.

As two physicians pointed out, the term "biopsy" is a bit misleading since it often implies a minor procedure and a cone biopsy is surgery, albeit minor, in which a cone-shaped bit of the cervix is sliced off.[11] "Most gynecologists would rather perform a hysterectomy," they wrote, because of the skill needed to perform a good cone.

Kristie was twenty-seven when she had her first "cone." While her gynecologist had been pretty straightforward, telling her that scarring of the cervix might decrease her fertility, he hadn't warned her about the heavy bleeding that came a few days after the procedure, much heavier than a menstrual period, with large clots of blood.

The same bleeding happened when she had a second cone, her Pap smear having remained abnormal. Her doctor said he wasn't sure he'd do a third cone if it came to that. When her Pap smear remained abnormal, he referred her to a large university medical center.

*The doctor there "was the worst person I've ever encountered,"
Kristie recounted. "He said that he would never give a third cone to
anyone, he would give a hysterectomy and that was all there was to it."*

*Kristie attempted to get him to explain why and was unsuccessful;
in addition, the biopsy he took in the office was very painful.*

*"I asked a lot of questions, and I was very aggressive about why he
was doing each thing. I felt that I'd gone through the first two cones
trusting someone without asking a lot of questions, and now I was very
alarmed and disturbed. He became very angry at me, and I couldn't
figure out why. I said to him, 'You have a problem; I don't understand
the words you're saying.' I don't know if he hadn't encountered women
who asked questions, or if it was just his style, or what. I was so angry
about the whole encounter that I didn't pay the bill—and I wrote to him
explaining why I wasn't paying the bill."*

*After asking around, and doing some reading at a local library for
medical consumers, she found a sympathetic gynecologist at a large
cancer center. "His attitude from day one was that you can have as many
cones as you want, that his job was to protect my fertility," she said.
"But he also told me that after the third cone I'd never have another.
'You're going to have cryosurgery,' he said, 'because I'm never going to
let it get to that point. I'm going to watch you closely enough.' "* [Such
a conservative approach should be taken only when you are
certain that your doctor is skilled in treating precancerous conditions of the cervix—for example, in Kristie's case, at a well-
known cancer center.]

*The third cone was not followed by bleeding, although she did get
an infection. Fortunately, Kristie's Pap smear has been normal for more
than a year now, and she's beginning to be optimistic.*

Gynecologists disagree about whether having a cone will
cause problems with fertility and childbirth down the road. Is
there cause for alarm? Unlike U.S. doctors, Scandinavian doctors
have a good deal of experience with cone biopsies, because they
have used them to treat all phases of CIN for years now.[12] A
recent study from Denmark of 607 women who had undergone
conization concluded that these women did not have a greater
frequency of premature delivery compared to the general popu-

lation,[13] and other studies have found that there was no good evidence that infertility, spontaneous abortion during the second three months of pregnancy, or premature delivery could be correlated with previous conization.[14] Some gynecologists aren't convinced, however. One editorialist wrote: "In women who have not had their families or who have children and desire more, only enough tissue to make the diagnosis should be removed by conization of the cervix."[15]

Obviously, if your choice is between a cone or a hysterectomy, a cone is the better choice if you wish to have children. But you might query your doctor as to whether a cone is really necessary, and remind him or her that you don't want it to be any larger than necessary. And if you do become pregnant later, be sure your doctor knows you've had a cone—she might want to follow you a bit more closely.

IS A LASER CONE BETTER?

Some surgeons are now performing cone biopsy with a laser, which seems to cause less scarring and may possibly reduce bleeding.[16] One Swedish study, for example, showed that patients whose cone was taken with the laser lost only one-tenth as much blood during the operation and in the first hour after it.[17]

Does this mean the laser is better? It's probably too early to tell. "Doctors who use the knife swear by it; doctors who use the laser swear by it," said Dr. Daniell. As a result, you're probably better off choosing a gynecologist on the basis of his or her reputation for competence and willingness to adapt the treatment to meet your needs. If the choice were between one skilled in using a knife and one trying out a new laser, I'd take the knife! The technology itself isn't the issue, in other words; the doctor's skill is.

When Lyudmila was first told she needed a cone (see page 105), her doctor told her that it would require three or four days in the hospital and ten days' rest at home. He also told her she might start bleeding, which would require resuturing, and that if the bleeding didn't stop she might have to have a hysterectomy.

Not surprisingly, Lyudmila took notice when a friend who had a cone removed by laser was in the hospital one night and was back at work in two days, and she decided to go the same route as her friend.

Unfortunately, her experience wasn't nearly as smooth. Lyudmila had her laser cone as an outpatient (the way, in fact, that all cones are now performed), checking into the hospital in the morning and returning home that night. At first she felt fine. But by the second week she began to feel "crummy" and to bleed. Ten days after the operation her bleeding was heavy enough to resemble a period, something the doctor had said shouldn't happen. Although her problem cleared up right away, Lyudmila feels she may have traded initial complications for later ones. In the final analysis, the laser wasn't the panacea she had hoped it would be.

TREATMENT OF MICROINVASIVE CANCER OF THE CERVIX

In general, once the cancer has actually started to invade surrounding tissues, doctors recommend either hysterectomy or radiotherapy. But for a subgroup of invasive cervical cancer called microinvasive (in other words, cancer that has probably just started to behave as true cancer), many cancer specialists now recommend cone biopsy, since there is less than a 1 percent chance that such cancer has invaded the lymph nodes, the first step in cancer spread.

If you have such a microinvasive cancer, three criteria are important in determining whether you can safely forgo hysterectomy. First, the cancer should not have penetrated more than three millimeters into the surrounding tissue; second, the cone biopsy should remove all of the cancer and not merely take a slice out of the middle of it; and third, the cancer should not have invaded the blood vessels.

The three-millimeter limit was proposed several years ago by Dr. Creasman and his co-workers in the division of gynecologic oncology at Duke University Medical Center in Durham,

North Carolina.[18] While Dr. Creasman notes that at the time there was considerable criticism of their conservative approach, today cone biopsy is considered standard therapy for patients with zero to three millimeters of invasion.

In fact, Dr. Creasman and his co-workers suggested recently that some patients with up to five millimeters of invasion be treated by cone biopsy. Here there is an increased risk that the cancer may have spread to the lymph nodes, perhaps up to 8 percent. Dr. Creasman suggests that patients willing to take this increased risk can perhaps avoid hysterectomy.

Dr. Micha of California cautions, however, that if you have been diagnosed as having microinvasive cancer and want such conservative treatment, you should definitely be seen by a gynecologic oncologist or cancer specialist. "The criteria for microinvasion vary from place to place and you really have to meet very strict criteria to make it safe. If you're just off by one or two millimeters on the depth of invasion, or if there's a little bit of lymphatic invasion, or if there's blood vessel invasion, or if the volume of the microinvasive tumor is beyond a certain point, all those things mean it's a really dangerous cancer that has to be treated with a radical hysterectomy or radiation."

He noted that the definition for microinvasion tends to change about every six months, as more data become available, "so you really need somebody who's going to gynecologic oncology meetings constantly in order to know what's safe to leave in and what has to come out."

J. Taylor Wharton, M.D., of the M. D. Anderson Hospital in Houston, Texas, notes that in conservative treatment of microinvasive cancers "there's a small, indefinable risk that has to be determined." In an individual who is strongly motivated to preserve her uterus, he felt the risk was justifiable.

RADICAL HYSTERECTOMY

Once a cervical cancer is frankly invasive—in other words, has invaded surrounding tissues by more than three (or according to some gynecologists, five) millimeters or has other characteristics that indicate it cannot be adequately removed by cone biopsy—practically everyone would recommend that it be treated by either radiation therapy or radical hysterectomy. The ovaries do not necessarily have to be removed, however, since estrogen does not cause cervical cancer to grow and, at least in its earlier stages, cervical cancer does not tend to spread to the ovaries.[19]

A radical hysterectomy is a much more difficult operation than total hysterectomy, both for the gynecologist and for the patient, because lymph nodes as well as other tissues outside the uterus must be removed. The hospital stay is often much longer (up to three weeks), and women who have had this operation usually must have a catheter in their bladder for about ten days, compared to perhaps one day in women undergoing other pelvic surgery. Following removal of the catheter, a significant minority of women have no sensation in their bladder, resulting in urinary retention or incontinence.[20] Some may also tend to become constipated owing to the loss of nerve fibers to the rectum. For some of the smaller invasive cancers a more limited radical hysterectomy, known as a modified or type II radical hysterectomy, is sufficient treatment and can preserve enough nerve fibers to the bladder and rectum to maintain bowel and bladder function. Philip Di Saia, M.D., chairman of the department of obstetrics and gynecology at the University of California Irvine Medical Center in Orange, is an advocate of this procedure.[21] It's worthwhile to discuss it with your doctor if he or she recommends a radical hysterectomy.

Radical hysterectomy usually removes the upper one-third of the vagina, and postoperative scarring may result in further shortening. The vagina may be stretched through sexual intercourse, although sex may prove trying at first. If you start having sex too early after the operation, you may injure the scar; if you resume it too late, the vagina may be scarred shut, so be sure to ask your doctor for advice on the optimal time to begin trying.[22] If you don't have a partner at the moment, ask your doctor what steps you should take after the operation to make future sex as painless as possible.

Maureen's radical hysterectomy lasted five and one-half hours and it took her five more hours to come out of the anesthesia. She was in the hospital for two weeks and had a catheter in for ten days, "which I thought was marvelous. I can't imagine having abdominal surgery and having to get up four times a night to go to the bathroom."

Before she left the hospital, she had to have an x-ray to find out whether her bladder was working properly, and while she "passed" the test, she now feels at times that she has less control over her bladder than she used to, which has been embarrassing on occasion.

Maureen's scar runs from the pubic hairline up to and around the navel and stops a little bit above it. When she first saw it she was bothered by its lack of symmetry, but then she saw a TV show in the hospital that convinced her that her navel was probably better off for being bypassed. The surgeon didn't use stitches but staples, and "big long things that looked like the things you truss a turkey with. They weren't painful, and it wasn't at all painful when they took them out, which was a big surprise to me. They just looked disgusting." While at first her scar was very red, it has now faded. "I wear bikinis, I could care less," she says. "I've never been known for my modesty."

A radical hysterectomy can be performed through a bikini incision known as the Mallard incision, although this can be more difficult for the surgeon and takes a little longer. Dr. Micha reports that it is almost always the choice of younger patients— at least in southern California.

RADIATION THERAPY

Radiation therapy for cervical cancer is an alternative, but not a terribly good one, particularly if you are young. It destroys the ovaries and causes scarring of the vagina in about 80 percent of patients and also makes it impossible for the vagina to lengthen and lubricate during sex.[23]

"[Early] cancer of the cervix can be cured equally well with radiation or surgery," said Dr. Micha, "but in younger people one leans towards surgery because surgery can preserve the ovaries. Radiation therapy will knock out the ovaries so the patient will go through menopause at whatever age she's at and have to be on hormone-replacement therapy for the rest of her life. You can also avoid irradiating the bowel and bladder and all the other structures in the pelvis. And there's some evidence that radiation can cause secondary cancers twenty or thirty years later.[24] If you're dealing with an eighty-year-old, you're not worried about twenty or thirty years from now. In a twenty-five-year-old, you have to think about what will happen in twenty or thirty years. In terms of preserving the uterus [with radiotherapy], it's of no value at all in terms of reproduction."

DES DAUGHTERS AND CERVICAL CANCER

In the 1960s, a rare form of cervical and vaginal cancer was found in a number of very young women, and it was later shown that many of them had been exposed before birth to a synthetic form of estrogen known as diethylstilbestrol (DES), prescribed at the time to prevent miscarriage although it was shown in 1953 to be ineffective for this purpose.[25] The rare type of cancer that resulted is known as clear-cell carcinoma.

Luckily, the risk of developing this type of cancer has turned out to be small, at least so far. There have been about 500 cases overall, or about 1 cancer for every 5,000 women thought to have been exposed.[26] While a fairly large percentage of DES-exposed women show a greater rate of adenosis, a condition where excess tissue is seen in the vagina, this is no cause for alarm. According to Stanley Robboy, M.D., chairman of the department of pathology at the New Jersey Medical School in Newark, "an active treatment is often worse than the disease," and the presence of the excess tissue is probably in no way dangerous.

Many women know that they were exposed to DES during their mother's pregnancy and are being followed up. Of this group, only ten clear-cell cancers have been found in women with adenosis who originally tested negative for cancer. All of them are alive and well, reported Arthur L. Herbst, M.D., chairman of the department of obstetrics and gynecology at the University of Chicago, who originally made the association between these cancers and prenatal exposure to DES, showing that follow-up can save lives.

If you were exposed to DES, can follow-up also save your uterus? This is not an idle question, as DES-exposed women have a maximum risk of cancer between the ages of sixteen and twenty-two. Most doctors would say that to be perfectly safe you should have your uterus removed if cancer is found.

But a few DES daughters with clear-cell cancer have been treated conservatively.[27] Kenneth L. Noller, M.D., professor of obstetrics and gynecology at the Mayo Medical School in Rochester, Minnesota, has treated two DES patients by excising the tumor as well as the lymph nodes. If the tumor has not spread to the lymph nodes, then the uterus can be saved. Similarly, a group at M. D. Anderson Hospital in Texas headed by Dr. Wharton has used local irradiation to treat clear-cell cancers when they occur in the vagina and are at least three centimeters away from the cervix.[28] The treatment will not preserve fertility if the cancer is closer to the cervix because it will destroy the cervical mucus factor and can cause fibrosis and scarring that might close the cervix entirely. So far his group has treated over thirty patients this way. There have been five recurrences, and based on the characteristics of the cancers that did recur, Dr. Wharton believes that most doctors could now predict in advance which patients were likely to have recurrences and were therefore less suitable for the conservative treatment. Four patients have become pregnant, and two are now on birth-control pills because they've completed their families.

One unanswered question is whether DES daughters will show another peak in the incidence of clear-cell carcinoma as they approach the age when clear-cell carcinoma ordinarily reaches its peak, from forty-five to fifty-five. Another is whether they may be at a higher risk of squamous-cell carcinoma, the common cancer of the cervix discussed next in this chapter. So far, said Dr. Robboy, there is no evidence that they are at a greatly elevated risk.

Physicians recommend that all DES-exposed women, as well as women in this age group in general, have examinations once a year. If you know you have been exposed to DES, you should certainly tell your doctor if you haven't already.

LESSENING YOUR RISKS OF CERVICAL CANCER

Doctors now believe that squamous-cell carcinoma—by far the most common type of cervical cancer—is a sexually transmitted disease. More recently, they have come to believe that during sex, certain strains of a virus known as human papilloma virus are transmitted between partners and that this virus eventually may cause the cervical changes that become cervical cancer.[29]

Squamous-cell carcinomas are unknown in women who have never had sexual intercourse, and the chance of getting CIN or squamous-cell cancers appears to increase with the number of sexual partners a woman has had as well as the number her male partner has had. Some men seem particularly likely to give their partners cervical cancer.[30]

But while having more partners increases your risk of acquiring the virus, just as with any other sexually transmitted disease, you can get it from a single partner if that partner transmits the disease. And as with other sexually transmitted diseases, your risk will be significantly reduced if your partner uses a condom and somewhat if you use a diaphragm.

Unfortunately, many doctors don't seem to understand that a statistical correlation of cervical cancer and precancerous conditions with more sexual partners does not mean that everyone who gets it has been promiscuous or has had more than one partner.

While Kristie's difficulty in finding someone to do a third cone biopsy rather than a hysterectomy has already been told, she did even-

tually find a doctor with whom she was very happy. But she developed an infection about a week after the third cone, and when she came back to the hospital her gynecologist was abroad and she was seen by a resident. "He came in one day and said, 'I want to see you in private.' He immediately said, 'I don't know what kind of life you've led in the past, what kind of men are in your life now, but it's quite clear that cervical cancer is the result of having numerous sexual partners. I think you ought to change your life if you want to take care of yourself.'

"I was stunned and very upset," said Kristie. "I'm a very insecure person anyway, and he caught me at a point where I was down anyway and had no defenses."

While Kristie was in the midst of a divorce at the time, she had been monogamous for the previous five years when she had needed her first two cones.

Kristie believes that doctors should tell patients of the statistical correlation between more partners and cervical cancer, because it isn't well known and she wishes someone had told her. But she resented the patronizing, arrogant attitude of the resident. "It was presumptuous of him to tell me to change my life-style when he didn't even know what it was. He didn't even bother to ask."

But while the human papilloma virus now appears to be the primary cause of cervical cancer, other factors may also play a role in susceptibility to the virus.

Social class and living conditions, for example, seem to be related to cervical cancer.[31] Better living conditions, in fact, are thought to account for the fact that, despite the sexual revolution, the death rate from cervical cancer has been dropping in most developed countries, regardless of how often they screen with the Pap test.

Another factor that may interact with the virus is cigarette smoke. Women who smoke have a higher risk of cervical cancer, and this may be because they have been found to have more "mutagens"—chemicals capable of causing cellular mutations and perhaps cancers—in their cervical fluid.[32]

Birth control pills do not cause cervical cancer, but there is some evidence that they may cause precancerous changes to progress more rapidly to invasive cancer.[33] Many gynecologists believe, however, that it is not the pill itself but the fact that women who choose the pill tend to be those with more sexual partners and are therefore at greater risk for exposure to the papilloma (sometimes called condyloma) virus. Less controversial is the fact that barrier methods of birth control such as the condom or diaphragm reduce the risk of cervical cancer.

Maureen had neglected seeing her gynecologist for about three years, partly because she was afraid he would tell her that she had to stop taking the pill, which she had taken without problems for about fourteen years. "I just didn't want to deal with it, so I didn't go," she said, explaining that the local pharmacist kept renewing her contraceptive prescription.

When she finally did go at the age of thirty-eight, her Pap test showed dysplasia, and she went for a cone biopsy, which showed that she had invasive cervical cancer. Maureen researched the issue extensively and asked her doctor many questions. From her research she learned that perhaps one of the few times hysterectomy can be life-saving is for invasive cancer of the cervix. "Someone asked if I had considered alternative treatments like diet and I said no, that hanging on to my uterus wasn't worth risking my life. And I didn't have a lot of faith in brown rice." Her subsequent radical hysterectomy did not show any more cancer, so her chances of cure were excellent, and she had kept her ovaries.

While Maureen was probably correct about brown rice as an inadequate cure for invasive carcinoma, what you eat may help prevent cervical cancer. One recent study from Italy has shown that women who ate more than fourteen servings of greens or carrots a week had a lesser risk of cervical cancer than women who ate from seven to thirteen servings, who in turn had a lower risk than women who ate fewer than seven servings.[34] While the authors thought this was probably due to the beta-carotene, a precursor of vitamin A contained in both greens and carrots, they also entertained the idea that it might be due to some other element in the Italian greens. One study, of course, doesn't prove that eating greens will help prevent cervical cancer, but eating lots of vegetables has so many health benefits that unless you really hate them, eating a lot is not a bad idea.

HOW OFTEN SHOULD YOU HAVE PAP SMEARS?

The American Cancer Society used to recommend Pap smears once a year, much more often than they are recommended in most other countries. In 1980 the society changed its recommendations to bring them more in line with the rest of the industrialized world. Now, they recommend that all women over twenty and sexually active women under twenty have two Pap tests one year apart. If both are negative, then screening can be done every three years until the age of sixty-five.[35]

From a public health viewpoint, this recommendation is fine. If every woman had a Pap once every three years, the vast majority of cervical cancers would be caught in their precancerous phases, and hysterectomy as well as cervical cancer could be prevented. One of the problems, of course, is that poor women are the ones at increased risk, while upper- and middle-class women are more likely to get frequent Pap tests.

From an individual standpoint, is once every three years enough? Would a Pap every three years absolutely guarantee that you wouldn't be found with invasive cervical cancer?

The answer is probably no. For one thing, the smears are not very accurate. Doctors have no consistent technique for taking them and may allow them to air-dry, rendering them practically useless. Or the smears may be taken from an area where there are no abnormal cells. Even if the smear is taken properly, as we've seen, there is a great deal of subjectivity in interpreting the slides.

For another, while progression of precancerous lesions of the cervix tends to be slow, it may be faster in young, sexually active women. A British study found that 18 of 394 women with invasive cervical cancer had had negative smears within the previous six years.[36] Six of these women died. An Italian study found that 18 percent of women with invasive cancer had had negative Pap tests in the three years before diagnosis.[37] These may have been fast-growing cancers, the authors concluded, or the Pap tests may have been read wrong.

For all these reasons, particularly if you are young and sexually active, smoke, or take the birth-control pill, you might be wise to have a Pap test once a year.[38] Even if you don't have a Pap test at each examination, there may be other reasons to see your doctor once a year.

But remember that while Paps may occasionally pick up endometrial or ovarian cancer, they are specific only for cancer of the cervix. Therefore, abnormal bleeding or other symptoms should be reported to your doctor even if a recent Pap test was negative.

Summing Up

If you have an abnormal Pap test, you probably don't have cancer but are much more likely to have a precancerous change in the cervix known as cervical intra-epithelial neoplasia (CIN) or condyloma virus infection. CIN can almost always be treated either in the doctor's office with cryosurgery or laser, or in a minor surgical procedure known as a cone biopsy.

If you have a microinvasive cervical cancer, you may still be eligible for treatment with a cone biopsy.

If your cancer is truly invasive, then nearly everyone would recommend that you have either a radical hysterectomy or radiation treatment. While either gives the same cure rates, radical hysterectomy is often felt to be better if you are young because it doesn't destroy the ovaries as radiation therapy does.

If you were born after 1940, you may have been exposed before birth to diethylstilbestrol, which has been associated with an increased risk of a rare type of cervical and vaginal cancer. Luckily, the risk of cancer appears to be quite low, but you should be certain to tell your doctor if you were exposed to DES. Close follow-up—gynecological exams about once a year—could not only save your life but allow you to keep your uterus.

You can lessen your risk of developing cervical changes in a variety of ways. The main cause of such changes appears to be a type of human papilloma virus that is transmitted sexually, so moderating the number of partners you have, or using barrier methods of contraception such as condoms or diaphragms, will somewhat reduce the risk. Smoking increases the risk of cervical cancer; eating greens may reduce it.

If you are at high risk for cervical cancer, you may wish to have Pap smears once a year rather than once every three years.

Chapter 8

Saving Your Ovaries

"A favourite excuse for unnecessarily removing one ovary is that the woman has another one to go on with; the excuse could equally well be used to justify the abstraction of one of two shillings from another person's pocket. And the shilling left behind might be a bad one!"
Victor Bonney, M.D.

Sherry found out as she woke up from her cesarean section at the age of twenty-eight that her obstetrician had removed not only her baby daughter but a golf-ball-sized cancer from her pelvis. The obstetrician had kept her open much longer than it usually takes to perform a c-section as he tried to reach a cancer specialist. When he was unable to and the pathology report came back noting the cancer was totally encapsulated, or enclosed, her obstetrician had sutured her up without removing any organs. Her unusual cancer had arisen in tissue next to the ovary, but it was not itself located in the ovary. "You know how in a golf ball there are rubber bands inside and a hard plastic shell outside? Well, the rubber bands were my cancer," she said.

The next day, the oncologist, or cancer specialist, came to see her and said bluntly, "I wouldn't have taken a chance with that kind of cancer. I would have cleaned you out."

Sherry discussed this distressing announcement with her obstetri-

cian, who gave her some insight into the psychology of some oncologists. "Since oncologists constantly have to deal with cancer, their life is not the happiest," he said. "They're dealing with patients crying going in and crying going out. Their philosophy is 'Eradicate cancer. Clean her out. If we take out of her every organ that she doesn't need—and she really doesn't need those reproductive organs—how can she get cancer again?' And that's their mentality."

Because the cancer had been entirely encapsulated, Sherry was treated by close surveillance. But a year after her baby was born, when she was twenty-nine, a sonogram showed an unusual mass in her abdomen. Another test indicated it was growing rapidly.

Sherry rejected going back to the oncologist who had wanted her cleaned out, and instead went to one who had treated her mother for cervical cancer. "I just felt a sense of peacefulness with him that I hadn't felt with the other," she said. She also asked several doctors including her own obstetrician what they thought of the doctor she selected, and they all praised his level-headedness.

Her new doctor believed that, based on the tests, it would be necessary to perform a hysterectomy with removal of both ovaries and possibly chemotherapy in addition. While Sherry's husband said he wanted another child, Sherry, at the end of the meeting, told the surgeon, "I trust you, I have to trust you. I've made a choice, and now it's up to you. My preference is not to have everything taken out of me, but if it's cancer I want as much taken out of me as you can."

Her operation the next morning lasted four and one-half hours. The mass turned out not to be a cancer, just a "bizarre-shaped ovary, one of the weirdest he'd ever seen," Sherry recounted. The ovary was removed and sent to pathology, as were tissue samples from all over the pelvis, all of which came back negative.

Sherry emphasizes that the decision not to remove any more than a single ovary was made by her doctor, but she underscores the fact she had made every effort to find a doctor with a philosophy she could accept. "When you're out with the anesthesia, and everyone's saying, 'Oh, my God, she's got cancer, we've got to get rid of it,' and they're hysterical, somebody's got to stay calm," she said.

· · ·

Sherry's story shows how good communication between doctor and patient can help the doctor decide what to do even if something unexpected happens on the operating table.

Recent advances in medical knowledge have shown that it's sometimes possible to leave one ovary and the uterus with little risk even when cancer is found in the other ovary. This is particularly true for the types of ovarian cancers that tend to occur in younger women.

And while in the past the uterus has almost always been removed if both ovaries were, medical centers that practice in vitro fertilization are now recommending that young women in whom both ovaries must be removed consider keeping their uterus for possible implantation with a fertilized egg donated by another woman. It's now possible for women without functioning ovaries to carry a child to term, and about twenty children have been born to such mothers.[1]

Yet many surgeons take a cavalier attitude toward these important organs, often removing either one or both healthy ovaries. And surgeons who do not hesitate to remove healthy ovaries are, of course, not inclined to do much to save diseased ones. So before undergoing any surgery, it's very important to discuss with your doctor what he or she will do with your ovaries, healthy or not.

PROPHYLACTIC REMOVAL OF THE OVARIES

Particularly if you are forty or over and have decided that hysterectomy is the best solution to your medical problem, your doctor may try to persuade you to have your ovaries removed during the same operation, even if nothing is wrong with them. Formerly, doctors justified this approach by claiming that your ovaries would not function normally without your uterus, or that they might develop complications that would require further surgery. It has now been established that in most cases ovaries do function without the uterus,[2] and that reoperation for "residual ovary syndrome"—the medical term used to describe problems due to ovaries left in after the uterus has been removed—is rare.[3] The two reasons doctors now give for the prophylactic removal of ovaries are that the ovaries may at a later date become cancerous and that the ovarian hormones can be replaced perfectly by hormone-replacement therapy. We saw in chapter 2 that this replacement is far from perfect, although many women may find it adequate.

But it is true that ovaries may become cancerous, and with the exception of the two types of ovarian cancer most likely to occur in young women, it is a particularly bad form of a bad disease. Most cases are not discovered until the tumor is well advanced, and the chances of cure are about 30 to 40 percent. In fact, about three-fourths of women who develop ovarian cancer, according to Dr. Winston, are diagnosed in late stages of the disease where the cure rate is low.

For that reason, Dr. Winston, who is quite conservative about recommending hysterectomies, nevertheless doesn't like to leave the ovaries in when he performs one. "I've seen too many people with ovarian cancer. No matter what I do with them they don't survive. For that reason I think they're better served having the hormone delivered by pill rather than by ovary."

He concedes, however, that the risk of a healthy woman developing ovarian cancer sometime in her life and dying of it is relatively small, a little over 1 percent.[4]

While the overall risk is small, the risk for women who have their healthy ovaries left in at the time of hysterectomy is even smaller. This lower risk may be due to the fact that if the ovaries are healthy at the age when the uterus is removed, they are likely to remain so. Some authors have calculated that of every 700 women whose healthy ovaries are removed, only 1 would have developed ovarian cancer had they been left in.[5]

Some gynecologists believe that ovarian cancer tends to run in families and that if you have several relatives who developed ovarian cancer your risk may be as high as 50 percent.[6] They may therefore recommend that women in such families have their ovaries removed. But you should know that while this operation will prevent most ovarian cancers, it doesn't prevent them all:

some women have developed ovarian cancer even without ovaries.[7] Not all ovarian tissue is located in the ovary, and the cancers in these women arose from ovarian tissue elsewhere in the
abdominal cavity.

Other gynecologic cancer specialists doubt that ovarian cancer is inherited, and think that even if you have relatives who
developed ovarian cancer, your risk may not be abnormally high.
An alternative to having your ovaries out, they would say, is to
have your gynecologist examine your ovaries regularly, perhaps
with ultrasound. You might also want to ask about blood tests
that may help indicate the presence of ovarian cancer.

Since the decision to remove healthy ovaries is based mostly
on opinion, the age at which it should be done is also chosen
arbitrarily. Many physicians maintain that any woman having a
hysterectomy after forty should have her ovaries out, and some
hospitals reportedly have such a policy. As someone who has
passed the magic age, I find such policies shocking, and I wonder
how many men would consent to have their testicles removed
after the age of forty, testosterone replacement or not and risk of
cancer or not. One professor of medicine (not a gynecologist),
who prefers to remain unidentified, wrote: "Any advisory com-
mittee which recommends prophylactic bilateral oophorectomy
[removal of both ovaries] in women over forty who need hysterectomies needs considerable advice and education. Not only is it
medically unsound in my opinion, but it reminds me of the dic-
tates of the Germans in the 1930s and 1940s . . . in addition to
the moral implications of routine oophorectomy, estrogen replacement for twenty years is frightening."

Somewhat more logical is the policy of other gynecologists
to remove ovaries in women who are past menopause, which
occurs on the average at age fifty-one. But a few gynecologists
are beginning to question this policy too. Recent evidence indicates that even after menopause the ovary continues to secrete
some estrogen and testosterone, which is closely linked to female
libido.[8] "The human postmenopausal ovary is not the completely
inert, nonfunctional fibrous mass that many formerly thought it

to be," wrote Drs. García and Cutler in their plea for ovary preservation.[9]

Particularly bizarre, according to Dr. García, is the practice by many surgeons of removing one healthy ovary, supposedly to reduce the risk of cancer. "They usually remove the right one, so if the patient later develops pain on that side they'll know it's probably appendicitis," he said. "They usually stand on the right, which also makes it easier to do. Some say they remove the ovary that looks 'least active,' which may be a figment of their imagination. How can you draw conclusions as to what that ovary is going to look like two weeks hence?"

In fact, Dr. García has pointed out, women in whom one ovary has been left are at no lower risk of ovarian cancer than women who keep both their ovaries.

BENIGN OVARIAN TUMORS

Most ovarian tumors are benign, and gynecologists who find one on pelvic examination face a dilemma as to whether to operate at all. Most ovarian cysts are simply the cysts that result when an egg is released into the fallopian tube; the medical term for these is *functional cysts*. "The ovary normally contains cysts," says Dr. Chaitin, who has published studies of ovarian tumors. "That's how it functions."

Most cysts, in fact, go away on their own. But since there is no way to tell without operating whether an ovarian mass is benign or malignant, very large masses, or ones that do not go away spontaneously, may require surgery. There is a risk, which increases with age, that they will be cancerous. Unfortunately, this is an operation that is particularly likely to cause adhesions (see pages 67–68). So if your gynecologist recommends operating on an ovarian cyst, be particularly sure to discuss how high the risk is that cancer will be found or that the cyst could cause other complications by rupturing, and also determine whether the surgeon will be doing the maximum to avoid adhesions that could cause pain and compromise your fertility if you still wish to have children. To give you an idea of the risks, of 101 Swedish women operated on for ovarian tumors large enough to be felt upon pelvic examination, two-thirds were found to have either totally normal ovaries or functional cysts. During the following two years, 18 of these women were subject to further gynecological surgery and 17 women were infertile.[10]

The chances that nothing serious will be found are even greater if you are under thirty: in the Swedish study, 98 percent of women under thirty had either totally normal ovaries, functional cysts, or benign lesions including endometriosis. But one malignant tumor was found in a woman of nineteen, showing that such cysts cannot be totally ignored, even in young women. Recently, gynecologists have started aspirating ovarian cysts with a needle guided by ultrasound.

If your gynecologist decides the cysts on your ovaries are suspicious enough that an operation is necessary, be sure to discuss with him or her what is to be done if no cancer is found, since so many gynecologists take out ovaries for so little reason. Make certain that he or she will not remove an ovary just to justify having opened you up!

You should also discuss what will be done if cancer is found, particularly if you still wish to have children. As we will see below, two types of cancer, "borderline" ovarian tumors and germ-cell tumors, can be treated by removing the diseased ovary, leaving the uterus and other ovary intact.

"BORDERLINE" OVARIAN TUMORS

As we have seen in the chapters on cervical and endometrial carcinoma, some tumors resemble cancers in some ways and in other ways do not. In the ovary, such tumors are known as "borderline" tumors, or sometimes as tumors of low malignant potential. Sherry, whose story opened the chapter, had this type of tumor.

Such borderline tumors are more likely to be found in younger women and, in fact, are more common than out-and-out ovarian cancer in women of childbearing age.[11] Most frequently, women with borderline tumors are treated by hysterectomy with removal of both ovaries. But in a number of medical centers, cancer specialists are finding that patients treated by having only the diseased ovary removed do as well as those in whom everything is taken out, as long as the surgeon removing the ovary has done a thorough operation to search for tumor spread.[12]

Henry Tazelaar, M.D., a pathologist, and his co-workers at Stanford University Medical Center, for example, found that while patients treated by removal of only one ovary had more recurrences (either in the other ovary or elsewhere in the pelvis) than patients who had removal of the uterus and both ovaries— 23 percent as opposed to 7 percent—the recurrences were easily treated with further surgery or chemotherapy and the patients remained free of disease after additional treatment.[13] Some of them delivered children in the meantime.

The patients with a type of borderline tumor known as mucinous tumors—so named because they contain mucus—had an even better prognosis. No patient with a mucinous tumor had a recurrence, including those treated by removing only one ovary. In an earlier study, patients with mucinous tumors treated conservatively actually had a better survival rate than those treated more radically.[14]

If you have a borderline tumor in one ovary, many cancer specialists advise that you have the other ovary removed after you've had the children you want, since you do have approximately a 15 percent chance of developing a cancer in the other ovary.

GERM-CELL TUMORS

A number of ovarian tumors are known as germ-cell tumors, meaning that they arise from the same cells that give rise to eggs.

Enormous strides have been made in the treatment of these tumors in the past ten years, and chemotherapy can now totally cure most of these patients.[15] For example, of thirty-six patients treated at the University of California at Irvine from 1972 to 1983, only two died.[16] While ten of the earlier patients in this particular study were treated by removal of both ovaries and the uterus, in later years the surgeons started removing only the affected ovary and biopsying the other tissues. Chemotherapy, of course, has its own complications, but with its use, survival rates for germ-cell tumors have risen dramatically.

And if you are cured of a germ-cell tumor by chemotherapy, cancer specialists see no particular reason to remove your ovaries after you have had your children.

THE FROZEN SECTION

If you are operated on for a cyst or tumor, your surgeon will usually send samples of tissue to the pathology department for a "frozen section," or quick assessment of whether the tissue is benign or malignant. Even though this procedure, done while you are still under anesthesia, can be highly accurate for breast tumors, it may be less accurate for ovarian cancers, particularly in hospitals not set up to do them routinely.

As a result, says Dr. Chaitin, many pathologists prefer that physicians not base the decision to remove a woman's ovaries on the results of a frozen section but wait until they can do a permanent section, which takes at least a day. While this may mean that you will have to undergo further surgery later, it will probably give you a better chance of retaining your reproductive organs, according to several oncologists and gynecologists I talked with.

As Dr. Micha said, "I think all gynecologists know of cases where seventeen-, eighteen-, and twenty-year-olds have had everything taken out based on a frozen and then the final pathology comes back 'not a cancer,' or 'a low-grade cancer,' or a germ-cell cancer, or something where they could have preserved their fertility."

Dr. Micha continued: "Almost all these patients are under thirty years of age and they're healthy, so if they need a second surgery two weeks later [after the results of the permanent section are available] they will all make it through it."

Waiting for the final pathology report may also permit wider use of bikini incisions for most ovarian operations. "That type of incision is really not adequate for cancer surgery," said Dr. Micha. "But it's OK [for the initial operation] because 90 percent of these pelvic masses in young people are going to be benign. By waiting for a final pathology report, you can avoid most of those up-and-down incisions in young people and keep them happy with the bikini incisions, which I think is important cosmetically and psychologically."

If you want your doctor to wait for the permanent section, be sure to discuss this with him or her before surgery. You may have to support your points with some research, since many doctors have been taught that if any type of cancer is found, everything should be taken out immediately. The fact that only one ovary may have to be removed even if certain types of cancer are found "is new information, changes that have appeared in the last few years, and may not even be in many textbooks yet," said Dr. Micha.

KEEPING YOUR UTERUS

Traditionally, if both ovaries had to be removed, so was the uterus, which was seen as only a cancer-prone organ that would complicate estrogen-replacement therapy.

But test-tube babies are changing all that. While a uterus is still necessary to carry a child, now it is possible for women with no ovaries to be mothers. They will not, of course, be carrying their biologic child, and the hormones necessary to maintain the pregnancy must be given artificially. But such women can carry an embryo fertilized in vitro with their husband's sperm and an egg donated by another woman. So far the technique is highly experimental and is being tried at a handful of centers that work with more traditional test-tube babies, that is, those where the egg is taken from the ovary of a woman and reimplanted in the uterus of the same woman.

In fact, this approach is at least theoretically possible in older women who have already undergone menopause naturally, and Dr. Schinfeld refers to it as "menopausal pregnancy."

Dr. Utian, who heads the in vitro fertilization program at Mt. Sinai Medical Center in Cleveland, Ohio, counsels any woman who still wants children to sit down and discuss the issue with her gynecologist before she undergoes ovarian surgery. Even if both ovaries are so diseased that they must be removed, "that woman could carry a pregnancy, and although genetically the child wouldn't be hers she still would have gone through the whole process of pregnancy and labor and bonding with her husband. Although she's lost her ovaries, she essentially has her own baby. What with the difficulties of getting adopted babies,* it's a real alternative."

Summing Up

While many surgeons advise women undergoing hysterectomy, particularly women over forty, to have their ovaries out at the same time, you should make your own decision about this, weighing the slight risk of ovarian cancer, a very serious disease, against the need to take artificial hormones daily to prevent osteoporosis and other symptoms of an early menopause.

If you are undergoing surgery for any reason, you should discuss with your surgeon before the surgery what should be done with your ovaries if they are healthy, have some disease, or are cancerous.

The ovarian cancers most likely to strike young women are often adequately treated by removing only the diseased ovary, sometimes with additional chemotherapy.

Even if both ovaries must be removed, if your uterus is left in you may be able to carry a child later, thanks to new developments in in vitro fertilization.

---

* There are approximately 60 to 100 families wanting to adopt healthy infants for each infant available.

Chapter 9

Pelvic
Inflammatory Disease

Pelvic inflammatory disease is known primarily as a cause of infertility, and it is a formidable one. After one episode of PID, 10 to 12 percent of women will be infertile due to blocked tubes; after two episodes, 35 percent; and following a third episode as many as 65 percent of women may be infertile.[1]

But infertility caused by blocked tubes can sometimes be treated. Infertility caused by hysterectomy cannot, and in a small percentage of cases, PID will lead to hysterectomy, either by causing ectopic pregnancies in the fallopian tubes, by causing tubo-ovarian abscesses that can be life-threatening if they rupture, or by creating adhesions that result in chronic pain.

Neither preventive measures nor early treatment can always prevent tubo-ovarian abscesses or adhesions, but both can considerably reduce the risk. And if abscesses and adhesions do develop, there are conservative ways to treat them.

AN OUNCE OF PREVENTION . . .

The vast majority of cases of pelvic inflammatory disease are probably due to sexually transmitted infections.[2] The one exception is PID due to tuberculosis: If you saw the play *Talley's Folly* by Lanford Wilson, you may recall that the plot was built on the fact that Sally Talley was infertile because she had had pelvic tuberculosis as a teenager. But today tuberculosis is clearly the exception and sexually transmitted diseases the rule.

The type of birth control chosen can also make a difference. Barrier methods of contraception, such as condoms and diaphragms, especially when used in conjunction with spermicides, provide significant protection, and oral contraceptives reduce by about 50 percent a woman's risk of being hospitalized for PID, although nobody seems to know quite why.[3]

The IUD, which is basically now off the market, increases the risk of getting PID, with all IUDs increasing the risk somewhat and the Dalkon Shield increasing it tenfold. But don't be fooled into a false sense of security if you haven't used an IUD: one study of ovarian abscesses showed that two-thirds of the women involved in the study developed this serious complication with no previous episode of PID or use of the IUD.[4] However, IUDs did appear to increase the severity of the abscesses.

Since PID has been linked statistically to more sexual partners, you may find, unfortunately, that some doctors will blame you for having developed the disease, whether or not you've actually had numerous sexual partners.

In 1975, Jane, a special education teacher, using a Dalkon Shield, was admitted to the hospital because an abscess in her ovary had burst. She was found to have peritonitis, a dangerous inflammation of the abdominal lining.

"When I got to the hospital," Jane recalled, "I was told they had to operate. I asked the doctor, who was the chief surgeon, 'What are you going to take out?' I said, 'I'm not sure I want you to operate.' He said, 'If you don't let me do it you're going to die.' He gave me something to sign and I signed it: I had no choice. On the operating table I asked him a lot of questions, including why it was so cold. All he said was, 'Don't be a nosy woman.' "

The surgeon found that both tubes and one ovary were badly damaged, but he removed only the right tube and ovary. He told her husband later he had left in the ovary because she was under forty, but doubted they could ever have children. "You weren't planning to have children anyway," he told Jane's husband, a peculiar assumption which Jane thinks must have been based on the fact that she was thirty-three and using an IUD. She feels very lucky that the surgeon, with such an attitude, did not remove both ovaries and tubes.

The Dalkon Shield was not removed, and Jane asked whether it might have led to the infection. Her doctors thought not, but Jane had it removed sometime afterward anyway, because she wasn't so certain. When she asked what might have caused the abscess, she was told that no one knew for certain, but gonorrhea was often a cause. She asked to have a test for gonorrhea, which came out negative. Later, when she considered joining the lawsuit against the manufacturers of the Dalkon Shield, her doctor said that the fact she had asked for the gonorrhea test would be held against her in the courtroom, apparently because anyone who even suspected they might have gonorrhea could not be lily-white. "The doctor was not supportive," she said. "He took the attitude 'If you pursue this, we'll find ways of dealing with you.' "

Jane changed gynecologists, and when she decided at age thirty-seven to become pregnant she figured out by keeping temperature charts when she had the best chances and conceived immediately. She had no complications during pregnancy, and required a c-section not because of any damage but because her son was large. After looking at her tube and ovary the doctors told her it was "forgive the term—inconceivable—that I could have conceived," she said. "When my son was born we wanted to find the surgeon who'd said we'd never have children."

When Jane was investigating her case against the makers of the Dalkon Shield, she saw a lawyer who said that of 700 women he'd talked to, she was the only one who had been able to have a child. She has been unable to become pregnant again, however, and has learned that her tube is now fully blocked.

EARLY TREATMENT

Luckily, the majority of infections do not become as bad as Jane's. About 80 percent of cases of PID can be successfully treated with antibiotics.[5] One problem is that you may not know you have the disease. Early detection is possible, but often the presentation is so subtle and nonspecific that it's difficult for you or your doctor to make the diagnosis. If you show increased vaginal discharge or pelvic discomfort or chills and fever, you should see your physician promptly.

"Aggressive initial treatment, combined with prompt follow-up during recovery, usually prevents pelvic abscesses—the most serious acute complication of PID," wrote Dr. Andrew M. Kaunitz, assistant professor of obstetrics and gynecology at University Hospital in Jacksonville, Florida.[6]

Unfortunately, no one seems to know what the best treatment is, but two antibiotics together give better cure rates than one alone.[7]

One factor that influences cure rates is compliance. A study by the Center for Disease Control showed that women were somewhat less likely to be cured if they took antibiotics for less than 10 full days. Sexual partners should be treated, too, or you're likely to be reinfected.

One issue yet to be resolved is whether patients should be hospitalized. Currently, about one in four women in the United States with PID is hospitalized, and there are no good studies as to whether these women do better than those treated as outpatients, although it is generally recognized that if you are acutely ill you should be hospitalized.

There are two advantages to hospital treatment. One is that larger doses of antibiotics can be given intravenously. The other is compliance: some gynecologists feel that women cannot be trusted to take all the antibiotics prescribed, which puts them at greater risk for a smoldering infection that lingers on.

You may therefore have a better chance of not being hospitalized if you can convince your doctor that you understand how important it is to take all the prescribed antibiotics.

TUBO-OVARIAN ABSCESSES

Abscesses in the fallopian tube and ovary that develop as a result of PID can be life-threatening, a fact which has sometimes been used to justify the removal of both ovaries and the uterus. But while surgery may be necessary, and definitely is if the abscess ruptures, that surgery does not have to be hysterectomy.

Drs. Daniel V. Landers and Richard L. Sweet, of the department of obstetrics and gynecology at San Francisco General Hospital in San Francisco, treated 175 of 225 patients whose abscess had not ruptured with antibiotics alone.[8] The remaining 57 required some form of surgery although this was not always hysterectomy with removal of both ovaries and tubes.

Another team, Drs. William Roberts and J. Lee Dockery of the department of obstetrics and gynecology at the University of Florida College of Medicine in Gainesville, found that only 8 percent of their patients with unruptured abscesses required operation because conservative therapy had failed.[9]

While conservative therapy can preserve the uterus and ovaries, the chances for subsequent pregnancy are not good. Drs. Roberts and Dockery found that only two patients of thirty-nine treated conservatively became pregnant afterward. They noted, however, that if in vitro fertilization becomes more available, some of the other patients might in fact have a good chance of pregnancy.

If the abscess ruptures, as in Jane's case, the patient's life is threatened, and "you don't hesitate to operate—you operate right away on them," says Dr. Schinfeld. But even here hysterectomy is not always necessary.[10] Like ovarian cysts, abscesses can sometimes be aspirated with a needle.

In fact, it may not even be the best choice to save the patient's life. As Dr. Schinfeld points out, "There were studies twenty-five years ago that showed that the mortality rate was actually less if only the affected ovary and tube were removed, leaving the rest of the reproductive organs. When you're dealing with pus and bleeding and damaged tissue, to remove the uterus may be a very difficult and life-threatening procedure in itself," he said. "It's clearly the trend in this country to treat ruptured tubo-ovarian abscesses conservatively."

Unlike most of the other situations where hysterectomy might be performed, tubo-ovarian abscesses can be real emergencies, and here a woman is at the mercy of her surgeon. "It's hard when you're sick and need an operation to go looking around for other doctors and alternatives, and that's usually the situation that patients with tubo-ovarian abscesses find themselves in," said Dr. Roberts, now an associate professor of obstetrics and gynecology at the University of Florida at Tampa. "The type of operation depends on what the operating surgeon finds, but there is no question that it also depends on the orientation of the surgeon."

Should you find yourself in such a situation, he suggests that you at least tell your surgeon that you want to preserve your uterus and ovaries if at all possible, if this is important to you.

If you have had one episode of PID, you should know that you are at an increased risk of further infections, and you should be somewhat more vigilant if you develop any of the symptoms.[11] You should have time, though, to look for a gynecologist you can count on to treat you as conservatively as possible should you have further episodes. You will probably have a better chance of being treated conservatively if your doctor is connected with a university hospital. Here again, an infertility specialist might be a good choice as a gynecologist, even if you are not trying to get pregnant immediately. Infertility specialists would be competent both to treat the infections and to perform any surgery, says Dr. Roberts. In some cases, though, you may find that they want only to see patients who are trying to get pregnant.

Even if both of your tubes and ovaries must be removed, your uterus may be left if it's less damaged by the infection. That way you could still consider an in vitro pregnancy, discussed in the previous chapter.

ECTOPIC PREGNANCY

If you have had PID, you are six to ten times more likely to have a tubal, or ectopic, pregnancy.[12] This usually requires the removal of the tube involved, although some gynecologists are now able to save the tube in such pregnancies.[13] In the past doctors used to perform a hysterectomy after two ectopics, since without the tubes there was no way for the egg to be fertilized and to implant in the uterus. But now that in vitro fertilization is available, it makes sense for the ovaries and uterus to be left. You would thus be able to carry your own child, even though your ovum would have to be fertilized outside your body.

CHRONIC PAIN DUE TO ADHESIONS

About 18 percent of PID patients develop chronic pelvic pain, thought to be due to the development of adhesions, or scar tissue, in the pelvis. As we discussed in earlier chapters, such adhesions may also result from prior operations, or as we shall see in the next chapters, from endometriosis. Since adhesions due to all these causes are treated the same way, they will be discussed more thoroughly in the next chapter, on pain.

Summing Up

You can reduce the risk of pelvic inflammatory disease by not using an IUD, by use of barrier methods of contraception such as the condom or diaphragm with spermicidal creams, or by remaining monogamous.

If you develop signs of infection such as increased vaginal discharge or chills and fever, see a doctor immediately. Treatment is most effective if two antibiotics are used together, and you should take the entire prescription. Most PID can be effectively treated this way.

If you develop a tubo-ovarian abscess, you may need surgery, and some surgeons will try harder than others to preserve your uterus and ovaries. At the very least, tell your surgeon if future fertility is important to you. If you have time to look for a surgeon, your best bet would be to find a doctor connected with a university hospital, or an infertility specialist who is willing to accept you as a patient.

Chapter 10

Pain—Menstrual, Sexual, and Chronic

"Those who do not feel pain seldom think that it is felt." Samuel Johnson

When Monique was thirty-eight, she took a trip to California and Arizona and, upon returning, began to have excruciating rectal pain. "I thought, 'Well, it's all that hot Mexican food—it burns going in, it burns going out.' One month later I had it again, and I thought, 'It's not Mexican food this time,' and decided I should get it checked." She also had nearly constant pelvic pain. "I would feel like somebody'd taken a bottle of acid and poured it inside my whole abdominal area." After trying a few doctors, she found a gastroenterologist who realized she had endometriosis. And after trying a few treatments for endometriosis, she eventually opted for a procedure known as videolaserlaparoscopy. "It was as if he took two bricks out of my abdomen," said Monique of the doctor who performed the procedure.

Most of us have had pelvic pain at some point in our lives. For many of us it comes in the form of menstrual cramps, which we can deal with in a number of different ways, the most effective being the antiprostaglandins that came on the market in the

1970s. But if you have cramps that are so severe that antiprostaglandins don't work, have pelvic pain constantly, or have painful
intercourse that's not due to an infection, you may need something stronger. Don't rush into a hysterectomy for pain, though,
since hysterectomy may not cure the pain and may even make it
worse.[1] "Sometimes the best treatment is indeed hysterectomy,"
said Dr. Schinfeld, "but sometimes when you do a hysterectomy
the pain is still there. Hysterectomy is useful in relieving pain
only when the uterus is the cause of the pain."

Depending on the type of pain, you have a variety of options. The disease causing the pain may be treatable or you might
be able to wear a machine that transmits weak electrical signals
through the skin to block the pain. In some cases surgical procedures can be extremely helpful.

Monique's story at the beginning of this chapter illustrates a
precept of Roger Smith, M.D., chief of the section of general
gynecology at the Medical College of Georgia in Augusta, when
dealing with pain: "Your best bet is diagnosis."

Once the cause of your pain is diagnosed, treatments can be
better adapted to it, and you may perhaps be cured. But particularly for women like Monique whose pain is due to endometriosis, just getting the diagnosis itself may be a relief. Many
endometriosis patients have been told for years that their pain is
in their head, since the only way to know whether you have the
disease is for the doctor to look into the abdomen. Said one
endometriosis patient of the time before she was diagnosed: "I
would go over in my head, 'What am I doing to myself that I'm
emotionally causing this pain that's constant? The pain when I
go to the bathroom in the morning, am I causing that with my
mind?' I would think, 'Who am I? What am I doing?' The fear
was incredible."

DIAGNOSIS

The most common way to diagnose pelvic pain is by a procedure
known as laparoscopy, in which two or three tiny incisions are

made in the abdomen under anesthesia and a laparoscope inserted to look inside.

When should you have it? Obviously doctors will differ somewhat in their recommendations, depending on your symptoms and their philosophy. As a rule of thumb, you might consider requesting one if antiprostaglandins worked for you when you first took them but no longer do much for your severe cramps, since such pain could be a sign of endometriosis. Having pelvic pain in the same location for a minimum of six months is another reason to request one. Arnold J. Kresch, M.D., an associate clinical professor of obstetrics and gynecology at Stanford University School of Medicine, was able to locate the probable cause of pain in 83 percent of patients with such a history.[2] Waiting six months is a good idea, he wrote, since your pain may disappear by itself during this time and you'll save yourself a minor operation.

Dr. Kresch found that most of his patients had either pelvic adhesions (38 percent) or endometriosis (32 percent). He treated these conditions during the diagnostic procedure itself, and 70 percent of the patients said they felt much less pain afterward.

ADHESIONS

Most of Dr. Kresch's patients who had painful adhesions had had either pelvic inflammatory disease or previous pelvic surgery. Interestingly, some women are found to have adhesions when they undergo surgery or laparoscopy for other reasons, even though they have not noticed any pain. In Dr. Kresch's experience, these women without pain were less likely to have had surgery or PID. Another significant difference in the patients without pain was that their adhesions were loose, allowing the organs to move freely. In the patients who had chronic pain, the adhesions seemed to be gluing the organs down.

Dr. Schinfeld agreed that while adhesions are often related to pain, the relationship may be complex. "Chlamydia, which is a sort of silent disease, may form massive, massive, massive adhesions without a great deal of symptoms. On the other hand, it sometimes forms fine, filmy adhesions. I call them Saran Wrap adhesions, covering the ovary so it's almost like a hard-boiled egg in a Baggy. Some of those adhesions can be extremely painful."

Such adhesions can be lysed (cut through) at the same laparoscopy during which they are diagnosed. Dr. Schinfeld said he thought that if adhesions could be lysed via laser laparoscopy (see chapter 11 for a more complete description of laser laparoscopy), "I would think that there's an 80 percent chance or better that we would get improvement in the pain."

But Dr. Smith cautions that adhesion lysis presents two problems. "The first is whether or not the adhesions are the cause of the pain. The second is when you break the adhesions, you may form two more, one from each broken end.

"Not only may surgery not be directed against the cause of the pain, but you run the risk that the pain may not get any better and it may even get worse because of what you did."

Dr. Smith said, "My own bias, and what I teach the residents here, is that if you're operating for pain, you've got to be very sure that both you and the patient understand that you can't guarantee that you're going to be able to change it, to take out the pain, and there is a chance that the pain will actually be worse because of new adhesions that the patient may not have had before."

If you have decided on a laparoscopy for chronic pain, be sure to discuss prior to the procedure what is to be done if adhesions are found. Will they be lysed then and there, which could save you an additional procedure? What chance is there that lysis of adhesions will cure your pain? And will your surgeon be using techniques to help prevent the formation of new adhesions?

UNEXPLAINED PAIN

If no cause can be found for your pain, some doctors will think you must be neurotic and will refer you to a psychiatrist or a pain clinic. Pain, of course, can be made worse by psychological factors, and pain clinics and even psychiatrists can probably provide you with helpful ways to deal with your pain.

But unexplained pain is a very complex problem, and not enough is known to say for certain that it's all in your head. It has always been suggested, for example, that pelvic pain might be due to poor circulation in the pelvis, resulting in congestion. The capacity of the ovarian veins can increase up to sixtyfold during pregnancy, and changes in blood flow can also occur with environmental and emotional stress.

Recently an English team has provided some evidence that congestion could indeed be the cause of pelvic pain.[3] When Dr. R. W. Beard and his co-workers of the St. Mary's Hospital Medical School in London injected a traceable liquid into pelvic veins of women complaining of pelvic pain, they found that the liquid took much longer to disappear in the women with pain than in control women who had no pelvic pain. In the women without pain, who were in the hospital for another reason such as tubal ligation, the liquid disappeared very quickly, usually before twenty seconds and in every case before forty seconds. But in the patients with pelvic pain, the dye was still there at forty seconds and in some it persisted for up to five minutes, indicating a sluggish blood flow.

Since these variations in blood flow are sometimes related to emotions, Dr. Beard and co-workers suggested that psychotherapy or other ways of dealing with stress are perhaps the most useful ways to approach them.

TRIGGER POINTS

Once you've really exhausted all the diagnostic options, said Dr. Smith, you have to work on breaking the pain itself: "Many times the pain becomes the disease." Centers specializing in the treatment of pain can offer a number of treatments such as acupuncture and biofeedback. Unfortunately, however, pain centers have shied away from the pelvic organs, just as gynecologists have shied away from nontraditional ways of treating pain.

One gynecologist who has tried to adapt methods of treating pain elsewhere in the body, such as backaches, to pelvic pain is John Slocumb, M.D., of the department of obstetrics and gynecology at the University of New Mexico School of Medicine.[4]

Dr. Slocumb incorporates a neurological examination into the pelvic examination, applying pressure over various dermatomes (the area served by various nerves) until he manages to duplicate the sensation of pain that brought the patient to him in the first place.

This approach is based on the fact that all pain sensations are brought to the brain by means of nerves, and while the origin of the pain may be in organs such as the uterus or ovaries, it may also be in the nerves themselves. In his examination, Dr. Slocumb identifies a set of points, known as "trigger points," that are central to the transmission of pain sensations.

Alice, whose story will be told in more detail in the next chapter, on endometriosis, underwent such an examination and treatment with Dr. Slocumb. "He did an exam where he would touch various points on my abdomen, and the points were tender. When he examines, he's just pressing very gently with his finger. You can sense different sensations where there's a trigger point. When he identified a point, he would make a mark with a pen. He performs a vaginal examination that's very different from most vaginal examinations, where he's looking for the same sorts of points. Afterward, he made a drawing with the little x's."

After the points have been identified, he then injects them with a local anesthetic. The injection initially reproduces the pain, but after a short time completely blocks it.

One woman I talked to found the treatments extremely painful. "I've had children and surgeries, and I've never had anything that hurt that bad," she said. "I would sometimes pass out with them."

But Alice found that while she initially didn't like the idea of having needles inserted at the trigger points, she found it essentially painless. She also found it amazing how injections at different trigger points related to very specific feelings. At one point, she got the exact sensation of pain she was getting with her periods. "At another point I had very bad leg aches. At another, I got very hot and started sweating. At another, I got bad stomach cramps. At one point I felt I was going to be in tears."

The pain relief often lasts longer than the local anesthetic. Dr. Slocumb wrote, "The anesthesia of 4 to 6 hours became weeks, months, and in some cases years of relief." Of the 122 patients with abdominal pelvic pain so treated, 52.5 percent reported no pain at all after treatment and 89.3 percent reported relief or improvement in the pain such that no further therapy was required.

Cherri, whom we met in chapter 2, found that after her "successful" treatment for endometriosis—a hysterectomy with her right ovary removed around the age of thirty—she had not only considerable bowel symptoms and diverticulitis, but also chronic pain. A retailer, she had to quit her job. "I couldn't sleep, I couldn't eat. I was losing weight real quick. I'd lost about nine pounds." At night, the pain was so bad she wanted to vomit. The doctor sent her to a psychiatrist, but the psychiatrist said, "This is real pain and it's really severe and we really need to get you to someone else."

Cherri lives in a small town in New Mexico, and she eventually went to Albuquerque to see Dr. Slocumb. After about four visits, the pain began to disappear. In about a month it resumed somewhat, but not so bad. Cherri says that if her worst pain was a "ten" her current pain is about "three." She can now work part-time. "As long as I have a chair where I can sit down every once in a while, I'm all right."

Dr. Slocumb found that this form of pain relief was effective not only in patients in whom no abnormality could be demonstrated but also in those with ovarian cysts, pelvic adhesions, endometriosis, and fibroids. In chapter 11, we will describe Alice's treatment for endometriosis.

Unfortunately, said Dr. Slocumb, few people around the country are trained in this particular technique of treating pain.

Most gynecologists don't know how to locate the trigger points, and pain clinics are hesitant about performing pelvic exams. He has taught the technique to his students at the University of New Mexico School of Medicine, but most of them have set up practice in the Southwest. If you write to him, however, he will try to give you the name of someone skilled in the technique.[5]

OPERATIONS FOR NONSPECIFIC PAIN

If your pain is exceptionally severe, you might want to consider one of the surgical procedures that destroys the nerves that transmit pain sensations.

The traditional procedure of this type is destruction of the presacral nerves, or the nerves that supply sensation to many of the pelvic organs. It is most commonly performed for painful menstruation due to endometriosis, often in conjunction with other surgery. It is also sometimes done for painful menstruation without endometriosis, deep pain during intercourse, and severe backache associated with menstruation. A recent report of fifty such operations found they were 73 percent successful in treating painful menstruation, 77 percent successful in relieving pain during intercourse, and 63 percent successful in relieving other pelvic pains. Eighteen percent of patients so treated developed pain later, although none had a recurrence of their painful menstruation.

All the same, doctors don't seem to agree as to whether this operation produces severe side effects.

According to L. Russell Malinak, M.D., a professor of obstetrics and gynecology at Baylor College of Medicine in Houston, bowel, bladder, uterine, or sexual dysfunction is rare after this operation.[6] Mild constipation sometimes occurs. "The only effect on menstruation is to make it less painful," he wrote. "Pain during the first stage of labor may be partly or sometimes completely relieved after this operation."

Dr. García agrees. "They don't have painful periods, they

don't have painful labors. The patients themselves comment that these are pluses."

If the sexual dysfunction following hysterectomy may be due to cutting of the nerves, what would be the effect of cutting the presacral nerve? "I don't know that I have really explored that, although patients haven't come to me to tell me they've had a difference," said Dr. García. "It's a limited number of bundles that you cut."

Dr. Smith of Georgia was less keen about presacral neurectomy. "It's not without major problems. It can yield some fairly nasty side effects in terms of problems with bowel and bladder control, and problems of sensation. Presacral neurectomy is generally reserved for really chronic debilitating pain when no other therapy is available—as a sort of last resort."

Dr. Daniell said that in presacral neurectomy the surgeon may cut so many nerves that a patient may not be able to feel when she has a full bladder. One such patient, described in a recent paper generally favorable to the procedure, has continuous leakage of a small amount of urine requiring the wearing of a sanitary pad.[7]

One objection to presacral neurectomy is that it is major surgery. "Presacral neurectomy takes four to five days in the hospital and several weeks to recuperate," said Dr. Daniell. "It also has a large potential for postoperative adhesions. I haven't done a presacral neurectomy in five years."

MINOR OPERATIONS FOR PAIN

Dr. Daniell prefers to destroy only one set of nerves, those that provide sensation to the uterus itself and are carried on the uterosacral ligament. This operation can be performed through the laparoscope, requiring a smaller incision and a shorter recovery time. It is mostly used for women who have extremely painful menstruation, with or without endometriosis. It will also work in certain women who have pain during intercourse. "If a person has a fibroid and is having uterine spasms during intercourse, then that can be helped. That's pretty rare. Most people with pain during intercourse have other pathology that's not going to be corrected by cutting the nerves that come from the uterus. It's not useful for chronic abdominal pain at all," he said.

In endometriosis patients, Dr. Daniell says, the surgeon can see the nerves well enough to cut them in about 80 percent of patients, and of these, at least 50 percent get good results. If the surgeon does a good job, the results seem to last indefinitely, said Dr. Daniell, or at least four or five years, which is as long as he has been performing them. "It's minor, outpatient, same-day surgery. It doesn't cause adhesions or scars." The procedure, however, is controversial among gynecologists; some claim their results aren't this good.

One *potential* side effect of this operation is that by abolishing the sensation of uterine contractions, some of the pleasure of orgasm might be lessened. While Dr. Daniell says the procedure doesn't have any effect on a woman's perception of orgasm, this may be because his patients were having so much pain before the operation that they really didn't care.

When used by someone like Dr. Daniell, who believes that women should be informed about what is happening to them and that procedures should be done only when there is a reason for them, destruction of the uterosacral ligament undoubtedly helps more than it hurts. The danger is that some doctors may use the procedure indiscriminately, whether or not pain is your problem. If, for example, you aren't having much pain but are having a laparoscopy to determine why you are infertile, you probably wouldn't want the procedure performed. As with all medical procedures, be sure to talk to your doctor beforehand to make sure both of you agree exactly what is to be done and why.

PAINFUL INTERCOURSE

The most common cause of painful intercourse is a vaginal infection. But if you have deep pain during intercourse that isn't due to an infection, it might be due to a tilted uterus. Sometimes the uterus begins to come loose from its moorings, and may either prolapse, coming out through the vagina (see chapter 12), or tilt. A tilted uterus is nothing to worry about if you have no symptoms, but it can sometimes produce pain during intercourse, as the penis pushes against it. The technical term for pain during intercourse is dyspareunia, and Dr. Daniell calls this situation "collision dyspareunia." Such patients respond very well to a procedure in which the uterus is placed back where it normally should be; this is known as a suspension and can be performed during a laparoscopy.

Dr. Stephen Gordon of Shallowford Community Hospital in Atlanta has tried the procedure in women with a tipped uterus and pain during intercourse but without other disease.[8] He reported that seventy-four of seventy-seven women who underwent the procedure had a reduction in their pain during intercourse.

But a potential problem with this procedure is that if the ligaments are weak in the first place, they may not hold up when suspended. Dr. Daniell suggests that such suspensions fall in about half of women after six months to a year. "It can be redone —but if it falls because of weak ligaments, it's probably not going to hold up much longer anyway."

This procedure will not work, said Dr. Daniell, if your painful intercourse is due to scar tissue, endometriosis, or fibroids.

NONSURGICAL TREATMENTS FOR CRAMPS

At the beginning of the chapter I mentioned that while the vast majority of us suffer cramps at one time or another, for most of us the antiprostaglandins (such as Anaprox or Advil) are all we need. Birth-control pills are also very effective in relieving menstrual pain, a fact you might consider when you choose a birth-control method.

But if you are one of the few women who can't take the antiprostaglandins because they make you feel sick to your stomach, or if you just don't like the idea of taking pills, there's still another option.

This is TENS, or transcutaneous electrical nerve stimulation. In TENS, electrical currents are applied to the skin by means of a gadget a little larger than a cigarette pack, which can be worn under the clothes. One Scandinavian study found TENS stimulation about as effective as the antiprostaglandins for the treatment of menstrual cramps.[9] The gadget costs several hundred dollars, so you probably should try it before you buy one, and they can be bought only on prescription. You might check with a pain clinic in your area for further information, since TENS stimulation is used in a wide variety of types of pain other than menstrual cramps, such as chronic back pain.

"For someone who faces menstrual pain month after month and can't take medication for whatever reason, it's an alternative therapy that's certainly worth doing," said Dr. Smith.

Summing Up

Hysterectomies are sometimes performed for pain, but while they may cure the pain, you run the risk that they will not and might even make it worse. A diagnosis of what's causing the pain can give you a better idea of whether hysterectomy will cure it—and may suggest a variety of ways short of hysterectomy to relieve it.

A laparoscopy can usually determine if the pain is due to adhesions or endometriosis. The adhesions can be cut and the endometriosis treated during the laparoscopy. The uterosacral ligament can also be cut, which is particularly effective for pain arising from the uterus. Deep pain during intercourse can sometimes be helped by suspension of the uterus during laparoscopy.

Injection of "trigger points" with a local anesthetic may help if you have chronic pelvic pain for which no cause can be found, or even if the pain is caused by endometriosis, fibroids, ovarian cysts, and the like.

Presacral neurectomy, in which the nerves that supply sensation to many of the pelvic organs are cut, is major surgery and sometimes produces major complications, but it can be used if you are in severe pain and other methods don't work.

C h a p t e r   1 1

Endometriosis

Yolanda, now thirty-one and a first-grade teacher, began having severe menstrual pain when she was about eighteen. Her pain was always associated either with her period or with ovulation. "The pain was usually bad the day before, and the first two days were horrendous. There was one job I actually lost because I was in so much pain I couldn't go to work and the boss said I couldn't take time off for 'just cramps.' "

At twenty-five, Yolanda eventually ended up in the hospital, where her right tube and ovary had to be removed because of the damage caused by a ruptured dermoid cyst. While the hospital record noted that endometriosis had been found during surgery, she was not told about the diagnosis.

Yolanda continued to experience pain after the operation, and she was also depressed. She finally saw a private gynecologist who, upon getting her hospital records, discovered she had endometriosis. She was eventually treated with videolaserlaparoscopy, which abolished much of her pain.

WHAT CAUSES ENDOMETRIOSIS

Endometriosis results when bits of the endometrium (inner lining of the uterus) break away from the uterus and become attached to other organs, most commonly the ovary, bowel, or bladder, but occasionally even the lung. Since it is the endometrium that bleeds in response to hormonal stimulation each month, each of these endometrial implants will bleed each month at the same time the uterus does. For example, the rare patient who has endometriosis in the lung may cough up blood each month during her menstrual period.[1]

The menstrual bleeding outside the uterus can lead to a variety of problems. Since blood causes adhesions, endometriosis sufferers may form large ones, leading to chronic pain and infertility. Since prostaglandins in the menstrual blood cause menstrual pain, the pain will be felt everywhere the endometrial implants and therefore the prostaglandins are.

A popular explanation of endometriosis is that it results from retrograde menstruation, or menstrual blood that backs up into the tubes and spills into the abdominal cavity instead of flowing out of the cervix into the vagina. A problem with this explanation, though, is that the majority of women, whether or not they have endometriosis, seem to have some degree of retrograde menstruation: laparoscopies performed during the menstrual period show blood outside the uterus in the abdominal cavity in about 90 percent of women whether or not they have endometriosis.[2] Obviously, some other factor is at work in endometriosis that causes the leaked menstrual blood to implant.

Endometriosis has been referred to as the career woman's disease, because career women often defer pregnancy, which retards the growth of the implants. For this reason, doctors often tell endometriosis patients to get pregnant as soon as possible, though they rarely consider how getting pregnant may affect the rest of their lives.

Yolanda's doctor told her she should have a baby. "You're at stage four, you have very severe endometriosis, you're probably infertile," he said. "If you don't have a baby now I'll have to put you on a drug that can cause serious side effects."

Yolanda agreed, and since she was able to feel when she was ovulating, she was pregnant within a few days. But she experienced some pain through the first four months of the pregnancy, and it resumed shortly after her daughter was born. Sometimes the pain was so severe she couldn't get out of bed to take care of her baby, who had to be cared for by her husband, mother, aunt, or friend.

By March 1985, she went on danazol (a hormonal treatment described in greater detail on page 87) because she couldn't stand the pain. "I went through all sorts of hormonal zigzagging, roller-coaster emotions, and moods. My breasts shrank considerably, and I'm very small to begin with." Five weeks after she stopped the treatment, an ovarian cyst, which had shrunk on the danazol therapy, started growing again. "The doctor told me, 'Have two more babies, then we'll give you a hysterectomy, we'll take everything out, we'll castrate you.' These were his words. I was appalled and insulted that he should say the word 'castrate' because no man in his right mind would tell another man, 'We'll castrate you.' He told me that after the hysterectomy I'd be fine. I knew that to be untrue."

Hysterectomy is often recommended as a definitive treatment for endometriosis, and women such as Yolanda are told they will be cured. Often they are. But if the ovaries are left in, some 85 percent of endometriosis patients will have recurrences after hysterectomy.[3] Estrogen-replacement therapy may also result in a regrowth of the endometriosis, although many endometriosis specialists believe it is less likely to occur if hormone therapy is started a few months after the surgery. A small proportion of women—about 5 percent—will have recurrences of endometriosis even if the uterus and both ovaries are removed and no estrogen replacement is given.[4]

Carole first found out she had endometriosis when she was twenty-four and had emergency surgery for a ruptured ovarian cyst. Even after the diagnosis, her severe abdominal pains were attributed to an ulcer or a spastic colon. "Because of my position as a production manager, they figured I was under a lot of stress," she said. She had surgery again, but was told that the endometriosis would most certainly come back. She would bloat so much that she could go from a size seven dress to a size seventeen in one day.

When she was twenty-six, she had a hysterectomy and had both ovaries removed, which she was told would cure her. Endometrial implants were taken from about fourteen feet of her intestines and from her stomach, but it was not possible to remove them all. Her doctors felt the remaining implants would eventually shrink because her ovaries had been removed and there would no longer be hormonal stimulation to make them grow.

"The doctor stressed to me, 'No estrogen replacement. I don't care what you're going through; I would never give you the estrogen." *Carole had no menopausal symptoms except hot flashes during the first week.*

But unfortunately her lack of menopausal symptoms may have meant that her body was producing estrogen anyway, and the pains didn't stop. In addition, she started to bleed from the vagina. She was eventually put on danazol, and experienced muscle spasms and memory problems. "I'd go to the store for something and I'd leave the money on the table and I'd have to go all the way back."

She went in for surgery again two years after her hysterectomy. Over 100 endometrial implants were cleaned out, and her bowels were unstuck from her vagina.

Now, a year later, "I feel great. I'm not on any medication. No hot flashes, no depression, no nothing." *She suggests that her own experience would have been easier if she'd had a baseline estrogen blood level test before surgery, and suggests that women considering hysterectomy for endometriosis ask their doctors about such a test because it will enable them to monitor their estrogen levels after surgery. She also thinks the gynecologist who refused to put her on estrogen replacement was correct.*

"One woman called me who'd had seven surgeries after her hysterectomy. I'd never turn around and say to her, 'You shouldn't be on estrogen'—I'm not a doctor—but I asked her, 'Just for my own curiosity, are you on estrogen-replacement therapy?' and she said, 'Yes.' "

Carole also advises women considering hysterectomy to be sure about their decision. "You can't undo it. If you do decide to go ahead, don't second-guess it afterward, don't turn around and say, 'I made the wrong decision.' Make sure you cover all avenues before you do it.

"Having a hysterectomy is a major thing, and I'm not going to say it doesn't bother me," *she goes on.* "But I say to myself that I'm luckier

than someone who's missing a limb, or confined to a wheelchair, or
dependent on somebody for something. That's how I get through it."

Lyle Breitkopf, M.D., director of the endometriosis clinic of
New York Infirmary–Beekman Downtown Hospital, often sends
endometriosis patients considering hysterectomy to Carole for
advice. He also strongly recommends that if you are considering
hysterectomy, you undergo counseling for at least six months
before having the operation.

When Monique, whom we met in chapters 5 and 10, was told her
pain and irregular bleeding were due to endometriosis, she was put on
danazol, which caused her to gain twelve pounds and do things like
"leaving the parking lot at work and driving down the wrong side of the
road."

She finally told her doctor, "I want a hysterectomy, and I want it
in February." By then, she was on the board of the Endometriosis Asso-
ciation, and two of her fellow board members in New York were doing
wonderfully well following their hysterectomies. But when she went to
the meeting of the national board, she met women who weren't doing so
well. Some had had such severe menopausal symptoms they had to go on
estrogen early and had had recurrences of their endometriosis. One was
having pain during intercourse because her vagina had been shortened.
"It seemed like it wasn't the panacea that some people had experienced
it to be." Monique opted instead for a type of laser laparoscopy
known as videolaserlaparoscopy, even though it meant flying from New
York to Atlanta to have it done.

LASER LAPAROSCOPY

The conservative surgical treatment of endometriosis consists of
removing the implants or destroying them, either by cautery or
more recently by laser. It's still not clear whether laser is actually
better than cautery, but gynecologists who use it are enthusiastic.
For example, Robert Breitstein, M.D., a clinical assistant professor of obstetrics and gynecology at New York University, has found

himself a convert to the laser, though he was originally skeptical about laser laparoscopy—"I thought it was magic, and magic doesn't work." Now he believes that laser is preferable to cautery because it can be controlled more easily. "There's more side dispersion [resulting in damage to adjacent tissue] with cautery. Using the laser you can be quite specific as to which tissue you destroy —specific to one-tenth of a millimeter. There's much less blood loss, less thermal damage, and fewer postoperative adhesions."

Dr. Daniell is also a partisan of the laser:[5] "Cautery works very well, but you run the risk of injuring the intestine. You occasionally get adhesions. There are some areas you can't cauterize, such as over the fallopian tube or bladder, because you'll burn them. But on other areas, cautery is very effective."

Since Dr. Daniell is skilled in the use of the laser, he prefers to use it both in laparoscopy and in laparotomy (a more extensive procedure). He cautions, however, that "destruction of lesions and adhesions by laser energy is a new, potentially advantageous surgical tool; however, it is as yet unproven regarding higher pregnancy rates or fewer complications, and the equipment is expensive."[6]

He also urges women seeking laser surgery to be certain that their surgeon is skilled in its use. "There are several questions you should ask your doctor if he proposes using the laser at your laparoscopy. What sort of training has he undergone? How long has he been doing this procedure? How many cases has he performed and what were his results? How much experience did he have with intra-abdominal laser surgery before he began using the laser through the laparoscope? Any competent surgeon should be willing to answer these relevant questions with honesty and frankness."

Since the laser has not been proven to be better than cautery, if you've found a gynecologist you like and trust who doesn't have a laser but proposes cauterizing the implants, you would probably be better off sticking with him or her. But if the only option your gynecologist offers you is hysterectomy and you consider that unacceptable, you might find it easier to locate a doctor skilled in laser than one skilled in cautery. You can obtain the names of gynecologists interested in the technique via the American Fertility Society, the American Association of Gynecologic Laparoscopists, and the Gynecologic Laser Society (see page 188 for addresses).

In most women the procedure, whether by cautery or laser, can be done via laparoscopy, in which the incisions are smaller and the hospital stay shorter than for laparotomy. In other instances—if there are endometrial implants on the intestine, for example—it may be necessary to perform the more extensive operation known as laparotomy, in which a longer incision is made and recuperation time is similar to that for operations such as c-sections.

One disadvantage of laser laparoscopy is that, if the endometriosis is extensive, the operation can be quite hard on the surgeon because he or she must bend over and peer into the laparoscope for long periods of time. Fortunately, the surgeon who performed Monique's operation, Camran Nezhat, M.D., a clinical assistant professor of obstetrics and gynecology at Emory University School of Medicine in Atlanta, Georgia, has developed a way for the surgeon in such cases to operate more comfortably, standing upright watching a video monitor. The operation is known as videolaserlaparoscopy.[7] With this procedure, Dr. Nezhat has taken on extremely severe cases of endometriosis, cases that probably no one else in the country would have attempted to treat conservatively through the laparoscope, partly because the procedure is so tedious. "You can hear the comments on some of the videotapes," said Monique, noting that Dr. Nezhat gives patients the videos he makes during their surgery. "Some of the gynecologists who are watching say, 'Oh, this case is so severe she should have a hysterectomy.' But Dr. Nezhat says, 'We'll do as much as we can.' And he did."

Besides vaporizing implants and adhesions, Dr. Nezhat usually dissects the uterosacral ligament, discussed in the last chapter (see pages 149–50). As a result, about 70 percent of patients have complete relief of pain.

· · ·

Monique went out to dinner the day after the procedure. She was back at work in a week. "I am not 100 percent better, but I am 90 percent better than I was before. I could not function before and now I can. And this technique is so easy that if I had to do it again I could. If I had to go back tomorrow, I would do it."

How long will laser laparoscopy last? "That's the $64,000 question," said Dr. Breitstein, noting that the technique does not usually cure the disease, although it buys time.

According to Dr. Daniell, following conservative surgery either by the laparoscope or by laparotomy, about 1 percent of patients will have recurrences in the first year, and by the eighth year 13 percent will. Can conservative surgery be repeated indefinitely? "Some patients have had two or three laser laparoscopies," said Dr. Breitstein. "Certainly you can have several. It's not a cure, it's another form of remission."

TRIGGER POINTS

Alice, a legislative fiscal analyst whom we met in the previous chapter, was thirty-four and unmarried when she had her laparoscopy for periods that were lasting three to four weeks with severe pain. The long periods and the pain were having a severe effect on her moods and emotions. "I was upset all the time. I work at a high-pressure job, and I couldn't afford to be feeling that way."

The laparoscopy showed widespread endometriosis, which wasn't treated at the time. Alice was advised either to get pregnant immediately or to have a hysterectomy within thirty to sixty days. While she does not particularly want children, "I didn't like the thought of having a hysterectomy—I'm not wild about operations because I think you can have just as many complications afterward."

Alice went to see Dr. Slocumb, whose work was outlined in chapter 10, on pain. While Dr. Slocumb has treated many patients in whom no cause can be found for their pain, he explained to Alice that he was beginning to think that the technique he was using for nonspecific pain might also work for endometriosis. He explained to her that pain itself might lead to chemical changes that caused endometriosis, rather than the other way around. In that case, the pain, rather than the endometriosis, should be treated.

Dr. Slocumb told Alice that he couldn't guarantee the results at all, but that if the treatment didn't work she might consider hysterectomy or other procedures later. "They were glad to get me, because I was relatively young and hadn't had much done," she said. "Most patients go to him as a last resort."

Alice took about three of the trigger-point injections, about one month apart, as described in chapter 10. She was also given antiprostaglandins to take for seven days before her periods.

After three months, her pain had abated and her periods were regular, lasting three to four days instead of the entire month. Her emotional and mental problems cleared up too, and she was able to think clearly. Alice continues the medications, but while she sees Dr. Slocumb every six months or so, she has had no more injections.

Without another laparoscopy, which she doesn't want to have, Alice doesn't know whether her endometriosis has been cured or whether only the symptoms have abated. Since her symptoms were her main problem, though, she really doesn't see the point of another procedure. "I couldn't be more pleased," she said of the treatment.

DRUG TREATMENTS

Nearly everyone I talked to, including physicians who specialize in endometriosis as well as women with the disease, agreed that surgical treatments, either via laparoscopy or laparotomy, are preferable to drug treatments. They made the following points:

- You should never be given drugs for endometriosis without a definite diagnosis, since the drugs given are strong hormones with definite side effects.
- The only way to get a definite diagnosis is to have a laparoscopy or laparotomy.

• Since the endometriosis can often be cauterized, removed, or lasered during laparoscopy, laparoscopy should be your first treatment, and may indeed be all the treatment you need. You would therefore be wise, if you suspect you have endometriosis but haven't yet had a laparoscopy, to find a surgeon who will be able to treat your endometriosis during your diagnostic laparoscopy, saving you further treatment, at least for a while.

Nevertheless, there are times when drug treatment may help you, for example, if your endometriosis was not treated when it was first diagnosed, if you have a recurrence after diagnosis, or sometimes in preparation for surgery, when treatment can make the implants easier to remove.

Since estrogen causes endometriosis to grow, all drug treatments for the disease use hormones to counteract estrogen, creating either a pseudopregnancy, where the estrogen is opposed by progestagen, or a pseudomenopause, where estrogen secretion is stopped or greatly decreased.

Real pregnancy and real menopause also work. You may be told to "get pregnant" as Yolanda and Alice were, but Dr. Breitstein admits that "the time-honored approach of telling patients to get pregnant is ridiculous"—unless, of course, you are ready to start your family anyway.

However, you may want to consider pseudopregnancy, created by taking birth-control pills continuously, instead of the usual cycle of three weeks on and one week off. Taking birth-control pills in the usual cycle is not considered as effective a treatment as taking them continuously, but it should slow the progress of the disease somewhat, and might be appropriate if your disease is mild.

Pseudomenopause is created with danazol, or more recently with a new treatment called GnRH analogs. As we have already seen, danazol may help relieve the pain and help you get pregnant if you are trying to, but it is associated with severe side effects.[8] Nearly everybody gains weight on danazol, although most patients gain under ten pounds. Breasts often decrease in size, although most of the time they will return to normal after the drug is stopped. Depression, muscle cramps, acne, and hoarseness may also occur. At least one case has been reported of a woman whose lowered voice never returned to normal after the drug was stopped.[9] A few patients develop hot flashes, others a skin rash. If you are taking coumadin, an anticoagulant drug used to reduce the risk of heart attacks and strokes, you should not take danazol, since the two together can cause serious bleeding.[10] While these symptoms are all reported in the medical literature, absentmindedness is not, although several of the women I talked to had experienced it. "A person I know was on danazol three separate times and she had three separate auto accidents while she was on it," said Monique.

Still, gynecologists believe that there is a place for danazol. "If the woman's trying to get pregnant and having painful coitus —nobody wants to go through that—you might want to use danazol, because it does diminish the intensity of the endometriosis for a few cycles," said Dr. García. It may then be possible for her to become pregnant after the danazol is stopped.

GnRH analogs, which also create a pseudomenopause, may have fewer side effects. Eldon Schriock, M.D., and his colleagues at the University of California in San Francisco treated eight patients with severe endometriosis and pain with one of these drugs known as nafarelin.[11] Seven completed treatment, and all had a decrease in both their pain and their disease, as confirmed by surgery afterward. The disadvantages of GnRH analogs, which are expensive, have been discussed at greater length in the chapter on fibroids (see pages 54–75) In brief, they produce menopausal symptoms during treatment, and the symptoms of the disease will recur once the treatment is discontinued.

SUPPORT GROUPS

While researching this book, I attended some sessions of the Greater New York chapter of the Endometriosis Association.

While I don't envy endometriosis patients their disease, I do envy them the support system they have created for themselves.

The Endometriosis Association is more than just a therapy group; it is to some extent a political force. We've seen time and again in the case histories in this book that a woman told by a physician that she needs a hysterectomy often feels alone and powerless to resist. But it's possible in many cases to arrive at a better solution by getting more information and by talking through the problem with people who can help you find your own solution and don't try to force you to accept theirs. Such a helpful exchange of information goes on routinely at meetings of the Endometriosis Association.

I noticed that while the two gynecologist advisors to the association were obviously respected, their word wasn't taken as gospel. The gynecologists actually listened to what the women felt would help them instead of deciding arbitrarily what *should* help them and then considering the women ungrateful if they rejected it.

Could women with other diseases form similar groups? I'm not sure. Those of us with problems like fibroids simply don't suffer enough to be motivated to do all the hard work necessary to keep such organizations going. And one woman said that her efforts to form a support group for chronic pain sufferers weren't very successful because "we just sat around depressing each other." So, many women will continue to end up alone when the gynecologist tries to get them to agree to a hysterectomy they don't want. But we *can* form informal support groups by simply talking with other women who have had the same problem.

Summing Up

You should never be treated with drugs for endometriosis without a diagnosis, and the diagnosis can be made only by looking into the abdomen via laparoscopy or laparotomy.

If you suspect you may have endometriosis, try to find someone who can treat the endometriosis with removal, cautery, or laser if it is found upon laparoscopy. This may be the only treatment you will ever need.

If you have a hysterectomy for endometriosis, your endometriosis may not be cured unless your ovaries are also removed. Sometimes the disease will recur even if both ovaries are removed.

While destroying the implants is probably the best treatment, hormonal treatments may help, although the side effects are troublesome.

Particularly if you live in the Southwest, you might look into the trigger-point injections being used experimentally at the University of New Mexico.

Chapter 12

Prolapse—Return of the Pessary?

"In many women who have had a long labor, violent pains cause forcible prolapse of the whole womb; here almost the same thing happens as frequently occurs in wrestling-bouts and struggles, when in our eagerness to overturn and throw others we are ourselves upset along with them; for similarly when the uterus is forcing the foetus forward it sometimes becomes entirely prolapsed, and particularly when the ligaments connecting it with the spine happen to be lax." Galen, 130–201 A.D., quoted in Logan Clendening, Source Book of Medical History

Galen was talking about the acute prolapse, or dropping of the uterus out through the vagina, that can sometimes occur with childbirth. But the general weakening of the pelvic muscles that can occur in women who have given birth to many and large babies can in later life lead to chronic prolapse of the uterus. The uterus may drop into the vagina and even out of the vagina, hanging like a penis. It may drag parts of the bladder or rectum with it, resulting in involuntary release of urine during a laugh or cough, urinary tract infections, and constipation.

Hippocrates, the famous Greek doctor who lived four hundred years before Christ, used several methods to treat prolapse, one of which was to tie the woman to a ladder which was then turned upside down and shaken violently.[1] Today, prolapse is commonly treated by vaginal hysterectomy with additional repairs made in the pelvic floor as needed. Even conservative gynecologists agree that symptomatic prolapse is a good reason to perform a hysterectomy, not because prolapse threatens a woman's life but because it makes it unpleasant.

As far as sex goes, women with severe prolapse may complain, said Dr. Utian, that "it feels like nothing's touching sides," or "I'm not really getting any enjoyment out of sex, it doesn't feel good."

"That's because the muscles are so stretched out that there is quite literally nothing touching sides," said Dr. Utian. "If you do appropriate repair, which may or may not involve hysterectomy but usually does, that patient's going to say, 'Things really are much better, there's really a marked improvement.' In a well-planned repair, patients will turn around and say, 'This has made such a difference. I didn't think it could be like this any more.' "

If you have severe prolapse, questions of the more subtle sexual losses that might be caused by hysterectomy itself may be immaterial. "Sexual function is very badly disturbed when you're dealing with that kind of prolapse," said Dr. Utian. "Your sexual function may not be perfect after repair, it may not be as good as it was twenty years ago, but it's certainly a lot better than it was last week before the surgery." Childbearing is often not an issue either, since at least in Western culture, if you've had enough children to have prolapse you've usually had enough to satisfy your maternal needs.

But here again, while you may want a hysterectomy if you have severe prolapse, it is not the only option. And there are several points you should know if you are considering a hysterectomy:

- Prolapse is a condition of weakened tissues, and there is some evidence it can be prevented, and that mild prolapse can be reversed, either by Kegel exercises (see page 172) to strengthen the muscles of the pelvic region or by exercise in general. Surgery, on the other hand, cannot make weakened tissues strong, although it may help to shore them up. Removing the uterus will prevent it from falling down again, but the bladder, rectum, and vagina may start sagging again even after hysterectomy. Therefore, if you can treat your prolapse by strengthening the muscles, you'll be much better off.

- Surgical treatment is necessary only if you have symptoms that are bothering you. An operation "is rarely indicated unless the patient asks for it," wrote Drs. John D. Thompson and Herbert W. Birch of Emory University School of Medicine in Atlanta in 1981.[2] "Entirely too many operations are done in patients who are asymptomatic. Unfortunately, some asymptomatic patients may be caused to have symptoms by an ill-advised operation."

- More than many other gynecologic operations, repair of prolapse can be rather easily botched and needs a good surgeon familiar with the technique. While other operations on the pelvic organs such as abdominal hysterectomy may cause a loss in the intensity of orgasm, it probably doesn't make much difference whether the surgeon was exceptionally good or mediocre, since the loss in feeling is due to the operation itself. But with prolapse repair, a mediocre surgeon can narrow the vagina so much that sex is not only not satisfying but impossible.[3] "Prolapse operations have a poor reputation for preserving sexual function," wrote A. G. Amias, a consultant gynecologist at St. George's Hospital in London.[4]

How common are recurrence and sexual disability following prolapse operations? It depends to some extent on the surgeon, of course. One presumes that gynecologists who report their results in medical journals are sufficiently proud of their skills, and sufficiently prestigious in their communities, to be reporting some of the better results. One group of Dutch doctors reported that 10 percent of their patients in whom prolapse was repaired with hysterectomy experienced pain during intercourse after the repair.[5] This compared favorably with another published report, where the incidence was 20 percent.[6]

Even in the best surgical hands, prolapse will recur about 20 percent of the time. The Dutch team noted: "The restoration of function and alleviation of symptoms occur in about 80 percent of surgically treated patients. Unfortunately, as time goes on the number of patients with persistent good results gradually decreases. Genital organ prolapse tends to recur. Unfortunately, and far too often, the final result is a distorted vagina and a return of symptoms. Thus, surgery cannot be considered a panacea."[7]

For example, of the 181 patients examined between seven and thirteen years after the operation, 38 had a recurrence of their stress incontinence, or involuntary loss of urine during laughing or coughing. One of these patients had been completely continent before the operation. Six patients underwent a second operation, but in only 4 cases was reoperation successful. The number of patients showing "urge-incontinence," or loss of urine when the bladder is full, had actually increased following the operation. Cystoceles (prolapse of the bladder) recurred post-operatively in 30 percent of their patients, and rectoceles (prolapse of the rectum) in 13 percent.

Given the fact that hysterectomy is a less-than-perfect cure for prolapse, you may first want to look at some alternatives.

CAUSES AND PREVENTION

The uterus is normally kept in place both by ligaments that support it from above and from the sides and by the muscles in the pelvic floor. Gynecologists differ in their opinions as to whether the ligaments or the pelvic-floor muscles are more important in holding the uterus in place. In some cases of prolapse the ligaments seem to be at fault; in others, the pelvic-floor muscles; and in some cases, both.[8]

Delivering lots of large babies and having difficult labors are thought to be responsible for many cases of prolapse. White women appear to be more susceptible than black women, perhaps because their uterine and supportive muscles are genetically weaker. In addition, poor nutrition and muscular diseases may lead to prolapse. The estrogen deficiency that occurs at menopause may accelerate the weakening of the muscles.[9]

Episiotomy (cutting of the pelvic floor during childbirth to allow the baby to come out without tearing) has often been justified as a way to prevent prolapse, and the apparently larger frequencies of prolapse in England have been attributed to the fact that English doctors and midwives use episiotomy less frequently than U.S. gynecologists, and when they do they use a different type of episiotomy.[10] But a recent study reported by Drs. H. Gordon and M. Logue of Northwick Park Hospital in Middlesex, England, has shown that the strength of the pelvic floor one year after giving birth bore no correlation to the amount of damage that occurred during birth.[11] There was not even any difference between these women and those who had had cesarean section, or those who had not had babies at all!

When, however, the women were asked about the amount of exercise they engaged in—both postnatal Kegel exercises and exercise in general—highly significant differences were found. Women who had never had a baby but didn't exercise much had poorer muscle function than those who had torn their perineum during delivery but were exercising regularly.

In fact, women who engaged regularly in such forms of exercise as exercise classes, walking, jogging, running, swimming, dancing, and yoga had slightly better pelvic-floor muscle tone than those who did regular Kegel exercises.

KEGEL EXERCISES FOR EARLY-STAGE PROLAPSE

The Kegel exercises, described on page 172, have been so promoted recently as an aid to sexual satisfaction that most people overlook the fact that Dr. Kegel originally proposed them to prevent prolapse and to reverse it in its early stages. "Even if genital relaxation is moderately advanced," he wrote, "viable muscle tissue is still present and can be effectively restored." [12]

Among his patients, approximately 75 percent who were diligent in their exercises reported some slight degree of improvement within a few weeks, he reported. Numerous patients who had been scheduled for an operation to correct their prolapse were placed on the exercises for a few months in order to control their urinary stress incontinence, and when these patients were subsequently reviewed, their relaxation was found to have been improved to such an extent that surgery was no longer required. Even when surgery is still needed, Dr. Kegel wrote, doing the exercises before the operation can reduce the extensiveness of the surgery, which can increase the chances it will be successful. So if you are considering a hysterectomy for prolapse, it certainly can't hurt to try Kegel exercises first.

Kegel advocated using a perineometer, an instrument inserted into the vagina to measure the force of the muscular contractions, for twenty minutes two or three times a day. He also advised women to contract the same muscles without the apparatus five to ten times every half hour throughout the day, and to interrupt the flow of urine several times while urinating.

Whether you use a perineometer or not, be certain that you are doing the exercises correctly. You might ask your gynecologist to check to see that you are. An entire chapter is devoted to the correct way to do Kegel exercises in the book *The G Spot*, [13] and you may also find instructions in childbirth manuals. Briefly, it feels a bit like "pulling your tail between your legs," which causes the vagina to tighten and bring the anus forward. [14]

Gynecologists don't all agree that Kegel exercises can prevent or cure prolapse. Don Sloan, M.D., of New York Medical College, for example, says he often tells patients with moderate degrees of prolapse that if they are not diligent with them he may have to perform a hysterectomy a few years hence. But Dr. Daniell counters that "exercise won't reduce the falling of the uterus —it will just kind of keep things inside a little better." The ligaments that support the uterus from the top and the sides are made of smooth muscle, he says, which doesn't respond to exercise.

Gynecologists do agree, however, that they see many, many fewer cases of prolapse now than they did a few years ago, even though prolapse is still listed as the third or fourth most common cause of hysterectomy. Perhaps the declining incidence of prolapse is a consequence of having fewer babies, perhaps of the popularity of Kegel exercises as an aid to better sex, or perhaps of the aerobics craze.

ESTROGEN REPLACEMENT

Dr. García notes that muscle tone often deteriorates at the menopause due to lack of estrogen, and that estrogen will often restore muscular strength. He cites the case of a patient whose uterus was completely prolapsed through the vagina who was admitted to the hospital to have some sort of treatment, probably vaginal hysterectomy. The gynecologist replaced the uterus temporarily with his hands, and the swelling of the vagina was treated with tampons soaked in boroglycerine. The patient was put to bed and given estrogens.

"When we saw that patient after three days, that uterus wasn't falling out any more. She never had her surgery, and she continued to do well," Dr. García said. "Every patient may not do well with this approach, but it's an attempt that one should offer."

PESSARIES

Hippocrates described treating prolapse by raising the foot of the patient's bed and sponging the prolapsed uterus with cold wine until it reduced in size. Half a pomegranate soaked in wine was then introduced into the vagina to hold it in place.[15]

The half pomegranate has its modern counterpart in the pessary, an instrument that can be made in a variety of shapes and is worn like a diaphragm in the vagina to support the uterus. Most gynecologists seem to consider it appropriate only for "little old ladies" who are not sexually active or who are too fragile for surgery, but there is no particular reason that it could not be tried by younger patients and discarded later if inconvenient.

"I have hundreds of patients in whom pessary control is working beautifully," says Dr. Winston.

Interestingly, gynecologists I interviewed differed in their opinions as to whether sex was possible with a pessary in place. Several told me that sex was never possible with a pessary. Thomas A. Rodenberg, M.D., a clinical associate professor of obstetrics and gynecology at the University of Miami School of Medicine, says that while this is true of most pessaries, there is one exception, known as the ring pessary. Another type of pessary is inflatable and can be taken out for intercourse and reinserted later, which, he says, some women become quite adept at.[16]

One inconvenience of the pessary is that it must be periodically removed and cleaned, usually by the gynecologist, and the vaginal tissues examined for irritation.

"I find that pessaries, and the problems that result, are a bother to the patient," says Dr. García. "It's not easy for the patient to examine her vagina for irritation. They do have a sort of tube where an individual can look up into her vagina and examine it. If you go through with these elaborate precautions, then a pessary might be functional. But I find that the patients who have pessaries are not that willing to exert that much effort. They neglect them and get irritations. It's like having gingivitis [inflammation of the gums]. Gingivitis shouldn't occur in anyone with proper dental hygiene and dental care. But people are careless."

Longer neglect may result in the pessary's becoming embedded in the vaginal wall.

For most women, then, use of a pessary will mean periodic visits to the doctor. But while the pessary may not be the solution for everyone with prolapse, some gynecologists report that certain patients are so happy with theirs that they can be described as "pessary addicts." When a pessary is used for the right indications, wrote Dr. Rodenberg, "the result invariably, and with only an occasional exception, will be a patient who not only will be able to resume the activities of a normal active existence but will be extremely happy and gratefully sing your praises."

Dr. Rodenberg acknowledges that younger women usually opt for surgery after a while because the pessary is a bother.

The advantage of a pessary is, of course, that you can try it and see if you like it. If you don't, you can always opt for a hysterectomy later.

OPERATIVE TREATMENT FOR PROLAPSE

If you have symptomatic prolapse that doesn't respond to Kegel exercises but you still do not want to have a hysterectomy, there are a variety of operations that will shorten the ligaments that support the uterus, thereby raising it. Unfortunately, childbirth can undo the operation. "A woman with this procedure could carry a child, but most people would say she should have a cesarean section," said Dr. García, "so as not to disrupt these supports."

Very few younger surgeons have done this procedure, however. "You should ask them how many they have done. I can't say that I've done very many myself, because there are very few prolapses these days," said Dr. García.

Still another option, but only for the woman who no longer wants to have sex, is a minor surgical procedure whereby the vagina is partly sewn together, thus providing an excellent support for prolapse. "You can do this procedure in the office in almost ten minutes," Dr. García said, noting it would be appropriate in a ninety-year-old woman who's not sexually active.

Summing Up

If you have had a lot of babies, your uterus may begin to drop down through the vagina. This is not a dangerous condition and needs to be treated only when the symptoms become bothersome to you.

One treatment is the vaginal hysterectomy, with other procedures performed at the same time to repair the prolapse. This treatment sometimes—but not always—improves symptoms. It is extremely important that you find a very good surgeon skilled in this operation because a bad surgeon can so tighten the vagina that sex becomes impossible. Keep in mind, too, that symptoms may recur several years after the operation.

If you feel surgery is too drastic, the pelvic-floor muscles can be strengthened by estrogen therapy and by Kegel exercises or exercise in general.

Pessaries (gadgets similar to diaphragms that are worn in the vagina) may be used to hold up the uterus either temporarily or permanently. Most do not allow you have to have sex, but one type, the ring pessary, does, and an inflatable type can be taken out and reinserted.

If you have severe symptoms that cannot be corrected by exercise and you do not wish to have a hysterectomy, several different operations can be done in which the ligaments supporting the uterus are shortened.

Chapter 13

A Patient's
Bill of Rights

"In the end it comes to this: you can't practice Medicine. You've got to treat people. It's people who shape and direct the Medicine you practice. They're the ones who make the rules.

"Sooner or later you'll have to come around to giving them what they want. Or else you won't have any patients. . . . It's their bodies, after all. We don't own them. All we've got is a license to practice on them."
Morton Thompson, *Not As a Stranger (1954)*

When I was a teenager, I remember being told, "Be careful what you wish for because it's likely to come true."

As I grew older, I realized, of course, that this is not always the case.

But it could come true in women's health care today because the number of doctors in general, and of gynecologists in particular, is increasing to the point that many are worried that they will not have enough patients.[1] In other words, supply is beginning to outstrip demand.

One possible consequence, of course, is that doctors may try to increase demand by convincing us that we need more and more examinations and procedures of all kinds. We should therefore be vigilant and make sure that everything being done is being done for our benefit, not just to give doctors enough to do.

But another consequence of the oversupply of doctors is that patients in general, and women in particular, are in an excellent position to ask for—and get—what they want.

It is therefore crucial to define just what we do want. Technical competence in a doctor is obviously important. But we also want gynecologists who are able to ask us what our preferences are, who can tell us the risks and benefits of different procedures and treatments, and who respect our right to make our own decisions based on the facts.

Since many of us find ourselves intimidated by doctors, either because the doctor really is intimidating or because we have been conditioned throughout the years to be unassertive "good girls," I therefore propose a bill of rights to keep in mind when you are faced with a recommendation for hysterectomy, or indeed any other procedure. Points 3, 4, and 8 state rights that are legally yours. The other points are mainly of psychological value, although perhaps someday they too will be legally ours.

1. You have the right to have your questions answered honestly.
2. You should never be "talked into" a hysterectomy, but rather given an honest assessment of what it can and cannot do for your condition.
3. You have the right to hear of alternatives to hysterectomy, even if your gynecologist will have to refer you to someone else for treatment.
4. You have the right to choose from among the alternatives the treatment you feel is best for you. This is true no matter what your age or your ability to have children.
5. If there is evidence that your condition may be related to your life-style, you have the right to be informed in a nonjudgmental manner. That you may have partially caused your problem does not negate your right to choose the best treatment for you.
6. You have the right of access to your medical records. (This right has not been legally affirmed in most states. But some

groups are supporting legislation that would make it easier
for a patient to obtain records.)

7. You have these rights regardless of your ability to pay.

8. You have the right to change doctors if these conditions are
    not satisfactorily met. (But please, to help other women, let
    your doctor know *why* you are changing.)
    Good luck!

Terms That Occur Frequently Throughout This Book

Adhesion. The "gluing" together by scar tissue of internal organs and tissues. Adhesions often result from endometriosis or infections, and are a common cause of pelvic pain.

Androgens. Male hormones, one of which is testosterone. In women, the ovaries and the adrenal glands secrete small quantities of androgens, which may influence libido.

Dilatation and curettage (D & C). A scraping of the endometrium (lining of the uterus). A D & C can be performed for the purpose of abortion; it can also be done in order to obtain tissue samples to be looked at for evidence of cancer or of hormonal stimulation. The D & C sometimes has a therapeutic effect on abnormal bleeding. The endometrium may also be "sampled" in an office procedure known as endometrial biopsy.

Dysfunctional uterine bleeding. Abnormal menstrual cycles, a sign that ovulation is not occurring and that the normal balance between estrogen and progesterone has been disrupted.

Endometrium. The inner lining of the uterus, the part that bleeds during menstruation.

Estrogens. A group of several hormones, all of which cause secondary sexual characteristics in women. Estrogens are produced by the ovaries.

GnRH analogs (or LHRH analogs). These substances are similar to the luteinizing hormone-releasing hormone (LHRH), which occurs naturally. This hormone is also sometimes called gonadotropin-releasing hormone (GnRH), since scientists are not certain whether it causes the release only of luteinizing hormones (LH), or of follicle-stimulating hormones (FSH) as well. Together, LH and FSH are called gonadotropins. GnRH analogs are being used experimentally to treat endometriosis, fibroid tumors, and abnormal bleeding; they act by producing a reversible menopause.

Hot flashes. Feelings of warmth and flushing that occur during menopause or after surgical castration. No one knows the exact cause, although hormones definitely play a role. Men whose testicles are removed also have hot flashes; and estrogen therapy can greatly diminish them.

Hysterectomy, total. Removal of the entire uterus, including the cervix. Total hysterectomy does not mean the ovaries are also removed, although an oophorectomy (ovarian removal) may be performed at the same time as a hysterectomy.

Hysterectomy, subtotal. This operation, which removes all of the uterus except the cervix, is practically never performed any more in the United States. Some evidence from Europe indicates that subtotal hysterectomy may have fewer negative side effects on sexual response and on urinary function than total hysterectomy.

Hysterectomy, radical. Removal of the uterus plus other neighboring tissues such as lymph nodes, an operation performed for cervical cancer. A radical hysterectomy can be performed without removing the ovaries.

Laparotomy. An operation in which an incision is made in the abdomen.

Laparoscopy. An operation by which an instrument called a laparoscope is inserted through a small hole in the abdomen to allow the surgeon to see inside. A laparoscopy may be performed for diagnostic purposes only, or certain procedures destined to have a therapeutic effect may be performed at the same time.

Laser. An instrument using the energy of polarized light. Lasers are used in gynecology both to cut tissue, in place of a knife, and to destroy it, in place of cautery or freezing. A possible advantage of the laser is that it may do less damage to normal tissues than other procedures. Also, because the laser cauterizes as it cuts, it may be particularly appropriate for procedures such as myomectomy and cone biopsies, where bleeding may be a problem. Two types of lasers used in gynecology are the carbon-dioxide laser, used in a variety of gynecologic procedures, and the YAG (Yttrium-Argon-Garnet) laser used in laser ablation (destruction) of the endometrium.

Laser laparoscopy. A procedure, usually performed for endometriosis or for the lysis (cutting) of adhesions, in which the surgeon looks into the abdomen with the laparoscope and at the same time destroys abnormal tissues with the laser.

Leiomyomas. The technical term for fibroid tumors, benign tumors arising in the myometrium, or muscular middle layer of the uterus. Leiomyomas can occur on the outside of the uterus (subserous); on the inside (submucous) where they can sometimes be removed with a hysteroscope; or within the uterine wall (intramural).

LHRH analogs. See *GnRH analogs.*

Menorrhagia. Heavy bleeding during the menstrual period.

Menopause. Strictly speaking, this means the cessation of menstruation. Under normal conditions, menstruation ceases when the quantity of ovarian hormonal secretions dramatically diminishes. Surgically, the uterus can be removed without removing the ovaries, thus ending menstruation before the ovaries have stopped secreting hormones. A surgical menopause, therefore, will cause the cessation of menstruation but not necessarily of hormonal secretion, and will not necessarily produce symptoms associated with the menopause. Surgical removal of the ovaries is known as castration: this will cause menopausal symptoms.

Myomectomy. The removal of myomas, or fibroid tumors, from the uterus. This is usually performed through an opening in the abdomen.

Myomectomy, hysteroscopic. The removal of fibroid tumors through the vagina with an instrument known as a hysteroscope. Only submucous fibroids, the type that occur inside the uterus and are most likely to cause bleeding problems, can be removed in this way.

Oophorectomy, ovariectomy. The removal of an ovary. Bilateral oophorectomy means that both ovaries are removed; unilateral oophorectomy, that only one is. In the *Index Medicus* the heading through 1985 was *castration*; in 1986 it was changed to *ovariectomy.*

Progesterone. A substance produced by the ovaries in the second half of the menstrual cycle and during pregnancy. During pregnancy, progesterone causes the uterus to secrete glycogen to nourish the growing fetus. During a menstrual cycle in which pregnancy does not occur, progesterone acts to a certain extent as an anti-estrogen, opposing the stimulatory effect estrogens have on the buildup of the uterine lining.

Progestagens, progestins. Synthetic compounds similar to progesterone that have the same actions. They are used in birth-control pills and, more recently, in hormone-replacement therapy to oppose the stimulation to the uterus (and possibly to the breast) caused by estrogen. They are also used to replace progesterone when the body cannot produce its own due to a failure of ovulation.

Suggestions for Further Reading Before You Decide to Have a Hysterectomy

Coping with a Hysterectomy, by Susanne Morgan (New York: Dial Press, 1982). Susanne Morgan had a hysterectomy and bilateral oophorectomy at the age of thirty for pelvic inflammatory disease. In this book she recounts her experiences and those of other women. While the title implies that the book is for the woman who has already had the operation, *Coping with a Hysterectomy* should also be read by anyone who is seriously contemplating one.

All About Hysterectomy, by Harry C. Huneycutt, M.D. and Judith L. Davis (New York: Reader's Digest Press, 1977). This is the best of the books written by doctors about hysterectomy per se that I've come upon. While I feel that it minimizes the side effects of the operation, the authors at least recognize that almost any condition treatable by hysterectomy can also be treated by other methods. In addition, the book is gracefully written.

Menopause: A Guide for Women and the Men Who Love Them, by Winnifred Berg Cutler, Ph.D. and Celso-Ramón García, M.D. (New York: W. W. Norton & Co., 1985). Remember that if you have a hysterectomy, you are undergoing surgical menopause, and that if you also have your ovaries removed, you will have more troubling menopausal symptoms than if you underwent a natural menopause. So be certain to read up on menopause before you consent to have your ovaries removed. Drs. García and Cutler are not only among the most knowledgeable people in the world concerning female hormones and the hormonal changes of menopause, but they have been at the forefront in advocating a conservative approach to the female reproductive organs.

Menopause, Naturally: Preparing for the Second Half of Life, by Sadja Greenwood, M.D. (San Francisco: Volcano Press, 1984). This book is useful both for women who have had a natural menopause and those who have had hysterectomies.

Listen to Your Body: A Gynecologist Answers Women's Most Intimate Questions, by Niels Lauersen, M.D., and Eileen Stukane (New York: Fireside Books, Simon & Schuster, 1982). Although the title doesn't indicate it, this also is a book that talks about alternatives to hysterectomy.

Once a Month: A Guide to the Effects, Diagnosis, and Treatment of Premenstrual Syndrome, by Katharina Dalton, M.D. (Claremont, Calif.: Hunter House, 1986). While Dr. Dalton's advocacy of progesterone for premenstrual syndrome remains medically controversial, she has been in the forefront of the fight against hysterectomy.

Endometriosis, by Julia Older (New York: Charles Scribner's Sons, 1984). According to sources in the Endometriosis Association, this is the best book there is on the subject.

Consent to Treatment: A Practical Guide, by Fay A. Rozovsky, J.D. (Boston: Little, Brown & Co., 1984). This book contains a chapter on women and reproductive matters with a section on hysterectomies. The cost is perhaps prohibitive for personal libraries, but try to persuade your public or medical library to acquire a copy.

No More Menstrual Cramps and Other Good News, by Penny Wise Budoff, M.D. (New York: G. P. Putnam's Sons, 1980). For many years I wrote about the use of antiprostaglandins in the treatment of arthritis, but it wasn't until I read Dr. Budoff's book that I realized they could be highly effective for menstrual cramps.

Clinical Gynecologic Oncology, by P.J. Di Saia, M.D., and W.T. Creasman, M.D., 2nd ed. (St. Louis, Toronto, Princeton, N.J.: C. V. Mosby, 1984). This book by the two leaders in nonradical gynecologic cancer surgery is written for gynecologists, but the prose is graceful and the approach refreshing.

Men Who Control Women's Health, by Diana H. Scully (Boston: Houghton Mifflin Co., 1980). While not as practical as the other books on this list, Scully's book on gynecologic training will help you understand how and why gynecologists think and act the way they do.

The G Spot: And Other Recent Discoveries About Human Sexuality, by Alice K. Ladas, Beverly Whipple, and J.D. Perry (New York: Dell Publishing Co., 1983).

And of course, *Our Bodies, Ourselves,* by the Boston Women's Health Book Collective, rev. 2nd ed. (New York: Simon & Schuster, 1976). An expanded edition, *The New Our Bodies, Ourselves,* was published by Simon & Schuster in 1985.

Some Useful Organizations

Women's Association for Research on Menopause (WARM), 128 East 56th Street, New York, N.Y. 10022. A group that raises funds for research on menopause and also sponsors support groups.

Hysterectomy Educational Resources and Services (HERS) Foundation, 422 Bryn Mawr Avenue, Bala Cynwyd, Pa. 19004, (215) 667-7757. Nora Coffey established the HERS Foundation following her own particularly severe experiences following a hysterectomy. A number of women I talked to reported that she had been very helpful not only to women who had had hysterectomies but also to women wanting information about alternatives.

Endometriosis Association, U.S.–Canada Headquarters, P.O. Box 92187, Milwaukee, Wis. 53202. A must if you have been diagnosed as having endometriosis, but also useful if you have experienced irregular bleeding, infertility, or severe menstrual cramps or other abdominal pain that might be symptoms of endometriosis. A visit to the association before you have a diagnosis can steer you to gynecologists who may be able to treat your endometriosis during the same laparoscopy at which it is diagnosed, thus saving you further surgical or drug treatment—at least for a while.

DES Action National. East Coast office: Long Island Jewish–Hillside Medical Center, New Hyde Park, N.Y. 11040, (516) 775-3450. West Coast office: 1638-B Haight Street, San Francisco, Calif. 94117, (415) 621-8032. A national organization devoted to helping women who have been exposed to DES.

The following are professional societies that might be useful in locating a physician who will treat you conservatively. Remember, however, that you should always try to get a second opinion concerning the doctor, since membership in such a society usually indicates interest but not necessarily competence.

American College of Obstetricians and Gynecologists, 600 Maryland Avenue S.W., Washington, D.C. 20024.

American Fertility Society, 1608 13th Avenue South, Suite 101, Birmingham, Ala. 35256.

American Association of Gynecologic Laparoscopists, 11239 South Lakewood Boulevard, Downey, Calif. 90142.

Gynecologic Laser Society, 500 Blue Hills Avenue, Hartford, Conn. 06112.

Notes

CHAPTER 1. *The Hysterectomy Hype*

1. A. M. Walker and H. Jick, "Temporal and Regional Variation in Hysterectomy Rates in the United States, 1970–75," *American Journal of Epidemiology* 110 (1979): 41–46.

2. C. L. Easterday, D. A. Grimes, and J. A. Riggs, "Hysterectomy in the United States," *Obstetrics and Gynecology* 62 (1983): 203–11.

3. There have been no studies directly comparing hysterectomy rates in France and the United States. Several studies, however, have indicated that the hysterectomy rate in the United States is about twice that of England: a recent one is K. McPherson et al., "Regional Variations in the Use of Common Surgical Procedures; Within and Between England and Wales, Canada and the United States of America," *Social Science and Medicine* 15A (1981): 273–88. Another study, comparing hysterectomy rates in England and France, found that 8.5 percent of women between the ages of forty and seventy in France said they had had a hysterectomy, as compared to 13.2 percent of English women. P. A. van Keep, D. Wildemeersch, and P. Lehert, "Hysterectomy in Six European Countries," *Maturitas* 5 (1983): 69–75.

4. There are exceptions, of course, to the general rule of bad books by gynecologists. These are listed in "Suggestions for Further Reading," pages 184-86 of this book.

5. F. M. Ingersoll and L. J. Malone, "Myomectomy: An Alternative to Hysterectomy," *Archives of Surgery* 100 (1970): 557–62.

6. F. G. Giustini and F. J. Keefer, *Understanding Hysterectomy: A Woman's Guide* (New York: Walker & Co., 1979).

7. P. A. Wingo et al., "The Mortality Risk Associated with Hysterectomy," *American Journal of Obstetrics and Gynecology* 152 (1985): 803–8.

8. E. R. Novak, G. S. Jones, and H. W. Jones, Jr., *Novak's Textbook of Gynecology*, 9th ed. (Baltimore: Williams & Wilkins Co., 1975).

9. D. H. Scully, *Men Who Control Women's Health* (Boston: Houghton Mifflin Co.: 1980).

10. S. I. Sandberg, et al., "Elective Hysterectomy: Benefits, Risks, and Costs," *Medical Care* 23 (1985): 1067–85. This article quotes a statement that, based on 1975 rates, 62 percent of all American women will have undergone a hysterectomy by age seventy. Since the rate has dropped slightly since 1975, the percentage should now be slightly lower.

11. B. C. Richards, "Hysterectomy: From Women to Women," *American Journal of Obstetrics and Gynecology* 131 (1978): 446–52.

CHAPTER 2. *The Side Effects of Hysterectomy and Ovarian Removal*

1. P. A. Wingo et al., "The Mortality Risk Associated with Hysterectomy," *American Journal of Obstetrics and Gynecology* 152 (1985): 803–8; C. L. Easterday. D. A. Grimes, and J. A. Riggs, "Hysterectomy in the United States," *Obstetrics and Gynecology* 62 (1983): 203–12.

2. N. P. Roos, "Hysterectomies in One Canadian Province: A New Look at Risks and Benefits," *American Journal of Public Health* 74 (1984): 39–46.

3. H. G. Hanley, "The Late Urological Complications of Total Hysterectomy," *British Journal of Urology* 41 (1969): 682–84; P. Kilkku, "Supravaginal Uterine Amputation Versus Hysterectomy with Reference to Subjective Bladder Symptoms and Incontinence," *Acta Obstetrica et Gynecologica Scandinavica* 64 (1985): 375–79; S. A. Farghaly, J. R. Hindmarsh, and P. H. L. Worth, "Post-Hysterectomy Urethral Dysfunction: Evaluation and Management," *British Journal of Urology,* 58 (1986): 299–302.

4. J. Shaughnessy, " 'Enormous' Hole Left in Woman's Bladder," *Medical Post,* July 8, 1986, p. 27.

5. B. M. Hansen et al., "Changes in Symptoms and Colpo-Cysto-urethrography in 35 Patients Before and After Total Abdominal Hy-

sterectomy: A Prospective Study," *Urologia Internationalis* 40 (1985): 224–26.

6. R. E. Miller, "Role of Hysterectomy in Predisposing the Patient to Sigmoidovesical Fistula Complicating Diverticulitis," *American Journal of Surgery* 147 (1984): 660–61.

7. D. A. Drossman, "Patients with Psychogenic Abdominal Pain: Six Years' Observation in the Medical Setting," *American Journal of Psychiatry* 139 (1982): 1549–57.

8. A. B. Ritterband et al., "Gonadal Function and the Development of Coronary Heart Disease," *Circulation* 27 (1963): 237–51.

9. T. Gordon et al., "Menopause and Coronary Heart Disease: The Framingham Study," *Annals of Internal Medicine* 89 (1978): 157–61.

10. L. Rosenberg et al., "Early Menopause and the Risk of Myocardial Infarction," *American Journal of Obstetrics and Gynecology* 139 (1981): 47–51.

11. J. Biró, "The Utero-Pituitary Axis: Influence of Nonsteroidal Uterine Factors on the Anterior Pituitary," thesis, Stockholm, 1983. Mimeo.

12. U. S. Department of Health and Human Services, National Center for Health Statistics, *Reproductive Impairments Among Married Couples: United States,* prepared by W. D. Mosher and W. F. Pratt (Washington, D.C.: Government Printing Office, 1982). A letter from W. F. Pratt explained that of couples who had been sterilized for medical reasons, two-thirds were sterile because the wives had had hysterectomies.

13. W. R. Greer, "The Adoption Market: A Variety of Options," *New York Times,* June 26, 1986, p. C1.

14. D. H. Richards, "Depression After Hysterectomy," *Lancet,* August 25, 1973, pp. 430–33; D. H. Richards, "A Post-Hysterectomy Syndrome," *Lancet,* October 26, 1974, pp. 983–85.

15. C. E. Vincent et al., "Some Marital-Sexual Concomitants of Carcinoma of the Cervix," *Southern Medical Journal* 68 (1975): 552–58.

16. N. B. Kaltreider, A. Wallace, and M. J. Horowitz, "A Field Study of the Stress Response Syndrome: Young Women After Hysterectomy," *Journal of the American Medical Association* 242 (1979): 1499–1503.

17. M. Steiner and D. R. Aleksandrowicz, "Psychiatric Sequelae to Gynaecological Operations," *Israel Annals of Psychiatry and Related Disciplines* 8 (1970): 186–92.

18. M. M. Seibel, "Sexual Function in Women with Pelvic Malignancy," in *Progress in Gynecology,* vol. 7, ed. Melvin L. Taymor and James H. Nelson, Jr. (New York: Grune & Stratton, 1983).

19. A. G. Amias, "Sexual Life After Gynaecological Operations—II," *British Medical Journal* 1975, 2, 680–81.

20. F. Hals, "Consensual Sex Can Result in Vaginal Tears," *Medical Post*, December 10, 1985.

21. Donahue Transcript #02285. Program aired April 22, 1986.

22. P. Kilkku et al., "Supravaginal Uterine Amputation Versus Hysterectomy: Effects on Libido and Orgasm," *Acta Obstetrica et Gynecologica Scandinavica* 62 (1983): 147; P. Kilkku, "Supravaginal Uterine Amputation vs. Hysterectomy: Effects on Coital Frequency and Dyspareunia," *Acta Obstetrica et Gynecologica Scandinavica* 62 (1983): 141–45.

23. P. Tunnadine, "Gynaecological Illness after Sterilization," Letter, *British Medical Journal*, March 18, 1972, p. 748.

24. L. Zussman et al., "Sexual Response After Hysterectomy-Oophorectomy: Recent Studies and Reconsideration of Psychogenesis," *American Journal of Obstetrics and Gynecology* 140 (1981): 725–29.

25. A. K. Ladas, B. Whipple, and J. D. Perry, *The G Spot: And Other Recent Discoveries About Human Sexuality* (New York: Dell Publishing Co., 1983).

26. J. Johnson, "Havelock Ellis and His 'Studies in the Psychology of Sex,'" *British Journal of Psychiatry* 134 (1979): 522–27.

27. L. Clark, "Is There a Difference Between a Clitoral and a Vaginal Orgasm?" *Journal of Sex Research* 6 (1970): 25–28.

28. R. C. Dicker et al., "Hysterectomy Among Women of Reproductive Age: Trends in the United States, 1970–1978," *Journal of the American Medical Association* 248 (1982): 323.

29. A. P. M. Heintz, N. F. Hacker, and L. D. Lagasse, "Epidemiology and Etiology of Ovarian Cancer: A Review," *Obstetrics and Gynecology* 66 (1985): 127–35.

30. R. B. Greenblatt et al., "Update on the Male and Female Climacteric," *Journal of the American Geriatrics Society* 27 (1979): 481–90.

31. B. L. Dennefors et al., "Steroid Production and Responsiveness to Gonadotropin in Isolated Stromal Tissue of Human Postmenopausal Ovaries," *American Journal of Obstetrics and Gynecology* 136 (1980): 997–1002; C. Longcope, R. Hunter, and C. Franz, "Steroid Secretion by the Postmenopausal Ovary," *American Journal of Obstetrics and Gynecology* 138 (1980): 564–68.

32. S. Chakravarti, W. P. Collins, and J. R. Newton, "Endocrine Changes and Symptomatology After Oophorectomy in Premenopausal Women," *British Journal of Obstetrics and Gynaecology* 84 (1977): 769–75.

33. S. M. McKinlay and J. B. McKinlay, "Health Status and Health

Care Utilization by Menopausal Women," in *Aging, Reproduction, and the Climacteric,* ed. L. Mastroianni and C. A. Paulsen (New York: Plenum Publishing Corp., 1985).

34. D. W. Pfaff and B. S. McEwen, "Actions of Estrogens and Progestins on Nerve Cells," *Science* 219 (1983): 808–14; T. Backstrom, M. Bixo, and S. Hammarback, "Ovarian Steroid Hormones: Effects on Mood, Behaviour, and Brain Excitability," *Acta Obstetrica et Gynecologica Scandinavica* 130 (1985, suppl.): 19–24.

35. Chakravarti, Collins, and Newton, "Endocrine Changes and Symptomatology After Oophorectomy."

36. F. W. Kraaimaat and A. T. Veeninga, "Life Stress and Hysterectomy-Oophorectomy," *Maturitas* 6 (1984): 319–25.

37. S.-E. Bjorkquist et al., "Carpal Tunnel Syndrome in Ovariectomized Women," *Acta Obstetrica et Gynecologica Scandinavica* 56 (1977): 127–30; M. Aitken et al., "Osteoporosis after Oophorectomy for Nonmalignant Disease in Premenopausal Women," *British Medical Journal* (1973): 325–28.

38. Rosenberg et al., "Early Menopause and the Risk of Myocardia Infarction."

39. P. A. Wingo et al., "The Risk of Breast Cancer in Postmenopausal Women Who Have Used Estrogen Replacement Therapy," *Journal of the American Medical Association* 257 (1987): 209–15.

40. W. H. Utian, "Effect of Hysterectomy, Oophorectomy, and Estrogen Therapy on Libido," *International Journal of Gynaecology and Obstetrics* 13 (1975): 97–100; L. Dennerstein, C. Wood., and G. D. Burrows, "Sexual Response Following Hysterectomy and Oophorectomy," *Obstetrics and Gynecology* 49 (1977): 92–96; H. G. Burger et al., "The Management of Persistent Menopausal Symptoms with Oestradiol-Testosterone Implants: Clinical, Lipid, and Hormonal Results," *Maturitas* 6 (1984): 351–58.

41. "Symposium: Adding Progestagens to Estrogen Replacement Therapy," *Contemporary Ob/Gyn,* September 1985, p. 237.

42. L. Fahraeus, A. Sydsjo, and L. Wallentin, "Lipoprotein Changes During Treatment of Pelvic Endometriosis with Medroxyprogesterone Acetate," *Fertility and Sterility* 45 (1986): 503–6.

43. Burger et al., "Management of Persistent Menopausal Symptoms with Oestradiol-Testosterone Implants."

44. H. Persky et al., "The Relation of Plasma Androgen Levels to Sexual Behaviors and Attitudes of Women," *Psychosomatic Medicine* 44 (1982): 305–19; B. B. Sherwin, and M. M. Gelfand, "Differential

Symptom Response to Parenteral Estrogen and/or Androgen Administration in the Surgical Menopause," *American Journal of Obstetrics and Gynecology* 151 (1985): 153–60.

45. "Symposium: Adding Progestagens to Estrogen Replacement Therapy."

46. R. B. Greenblatt and A. Z. Teran, "Sexual Dysfunction in Women: Does Testosterone Help?" *Contemporary Ob/Gyn*, July 1986, pp. 129–35.

47. "Symposium: Adding Progestagens to Estrogen Replacement Therapy."

48. J. A. Simon and G. S. diZerega, "Physiologic Estradiol Replacement Following Oophorectomy: Failure to Maintain Precastration Gonadotropin Levels," *Obstetrics and Gynecology* 59 (1982): 511–13; C.-R. García and W. B. Cutler, "Preservation of the Ovary: A Reevaluation," *Fertility and Sterility* 42 (1984): 510–14.

CHAPTER 3. *Strategies for Avoiding Hysterectomy*

1. G. Domenighetti, P. Luraschi, and A. Marazzi, "Hysterectomy and Sex of the Gynecologist," Letter, *New England Journal of Medicine* 313 (1985): 1482.

2. J. P. Bunker and B. W. Brown, Jr., "The Physician-Patient as an Informed Consumer of Surgical Services," *New England Journal of Medicine* 290 (1974): 1051–55.

3. J. Zimmer, "Would You Get a Second Opinion?" *M.D.*, September 1986, pp. 25–26.

CHAPTER 4. *Fibroids—the Most Common Reason Women Are Told They Need a Hysterectomy*

1. N. C. Lee et al., "Confirmation of the Preoperative Diagnoses for Hysterectomy," *American Journal of Obstetrics and Gynecology* 150 (1984): 283–87.

2. R. F. Mattingly and J. D. Thompson, *Te Linde's Operative Gynecology* (Philadelphia: J. B. Lippincott, 1985), p. 203.

3. Comment, *Obstetrical and Gynecological Survey*, May 1986, p. 319.

4. H. W. Jones, Jr., and G. S. Jones, "Myoma of the Uterus," *Novak's*

Textbook of Gynecology, 10th ed. (Baltimore and London: Williams & Wilkins, 1981), p. 427.

5. S. F. Cramer et al., "Growth Potential of Human Uterine Leiomyomas: Some In Vitro Observations and Their Implications," *Obstetrics and Gynecology* 66 (1985): 36–41.

6. E. A. Wilson, F. Yang, and E. D. Rees, "Estradiol and Progesterone Binding in Uterine Leiomyomata and in Normal Uterine Tissues," *Obstetrics and Gynecology* 55 (1979): 20–24; T. Tamaya, J. Fujimoto, and H. Okada, "Comparison of Cellular Levels of Steroid Receptors in Uterine Leiomyoma and Myometrium," *Acta Obstetrica et Gynecologica Scandinavica* 64 (1985): 307.

7. Jones and Jones, "Myoma of the Uterus."

8. R. K. Ross, "Risk Factors for Uterine Fibroids: Reduced Risk Associated with Oral Contraceptives," *British Medical Journal* 293 (1986): 359–62. See also letters that appeared in the *British Medical Journal* 293 (1986): 1027 and 1175.

9. A. H. John and R. Martin, "Growth of Leiomyomata with Estrogen-Progestogen Therapy," *Journal of Reproductive Medicine* 6 (1971): 49–51.

10. "Symposium: Problems Linked to Uterine Myomas," *Contemporary Ob/Gyn*, November 1983, p. 266.

11. J. A. Chalmers, "Uterine Fibroids," *Nursing Times*, October 28, 1976, pp. 1672–74.

12. V. C. Buttram, Jr., and R. C. Reiter, "Uterine Leiomyomata: Etiology, Symptomatology, and Management," *Fertility and Sterility* 36 (1981): 433–45.

13. G. Farrer-Brown, J. O. W. Beilby, and M. H. Tarbit, "The Vascular Patterns in Myomatous Uteri," *Journal of Obstetrics and Gynaecology of the British Commonwealth* 77 (1970): 967–75; M. S. Baggish, "Mesenchymal Tumors of the Uterus," *Clinical Obstetrics and Gynecology* 17 (1974): 51–64.

14. Ross, "Risk Factors for Uterine Fibroids."

15. A. E. Omu, I. J. Ihejerika, and G. Tabowei, "Management of Uterine Fibroids at the University of Benin Teaching Hospital," *Tropical Doctor* 14 (1984): 82–85.

16. Buttram and Reiter, "Uterine Leiomyomata."

17. V. Bonney, *Extended Myomectomy and Ovarian Cystectomy* (New York and London: Paul B. Hoeber, 1946).

18. V. Bonney, "The Technique and Results of Myomectomy," *Lancet*, January 24, 1931, 171–77.

19. Buttram and Reiter, "Uterine Leiomyomata."

20. L. J. Malone, "Myomectomy: Recurrence After Removal of Solitary and Multiple Myomas," *Obstetrics and Gynecology* 34 (1969): 200–203.

21. Bonney, "Technique and Results of Myomectomy."

22. D. S. McLaughlin, "Metroplasty and Myomectomy with the CO_2 Laser for Maximizing the Preservation of Normal Tissue and Minimizing Blood Loss," *Journal of Reproductive Medicine* 30 (1985): 1–9.

23. D. W. Briggs, "Abdominal Myomectomy in the Treatment of Uterine Myomas," *American Journal of Obstetrics and Gynecology* 95 (1966): 769–76.

24. Omu, Ihejerika, and Tabowei, "Management of Uterine Fibroids at the University of Benin Teaching Hospital."

25. N. Jeffcoate, *Principles of Gynaecology*, 4th ed. (London and Boston: Butterworth's, 1975), p. 424.

26. S. Roopnarinesingh, J. Suratsingh, and A. Roopnarinesingh, "The Obstetric Outcome of Patients with Previous Myomectomy or Hysterectomy," *West Indian Medical Journal* 34 (1985): 59–62.

27. R. S. Neuwirth, "A New Technique for and Additional Experience with Hysteroscopic Resection of Submucous Fibroids," *American Journal of Obstetrics and Gynecology* 131 (1978): 91–94; R. S. Neuwirth, "An Alternative to Hysterectomy for Fibroids," *Female Patient*, February 1979, pp. 54–57; R. S. Neuwirth, "Hysteroscopic Resection of Submucous Leiomyoma," *Contemporary Ob/Gyn*, January 1985, pp. 103–19.

28. Buttram and Reiter, "Uterine Leiomyomata."

29. A. J. Tiltman, "The Effect of Progestins on the Mitotic Activity of Uterine Fibromyomas," *International Journal of Gynecological Pathology* 4 (1985): 89–96.

30. T. Ziporyn, "LHRH: Clinical Applications Growing," *Journal of the American Medical Association* 253 (1985): 469–76; C. C. Coddington, "Long-acting Gonadotropin Hormone-Releasing Hormone Analog Used to Treat Uteri," *Fertility and Sterility* 45 (1986): 624–29.

31. R. Maheux et al., "Luteinizing Hormone-Releasing Hormone Agonist and Uterine Leiomyoma: A Pilot Study," *American Journal of Obstetrics and Gynecology* 152 (1985): 1034–38.

32. M. B. Kapp, "Prescribing Approved Drugs for Nonapproved Uses: Physicians' Disclosure Obligations to Their Patients," *Law, Medicine, and Health Care* 9 (1981): 20–23.

CHAPTER 5. *Heavy Bleeding—Regular or Not*

1. J. A. Fayez, "Dysfunctional Uterine Bleeding," *American Family Physician* 25 (1982): 109–15.

2. G. C. M. L. Christiaens, J. J. Sixma, and A. A. Haspels, "Morphology of Haemostasis in Menstrual Endometrium," *British Journal of Obstetrics and Gynaecology* 87 (1980): 425–39.

3. E. A. Claessens and C. A. Cowell, "Acute Adolescent Menorrhagia," *American Journal of Obstetrics and Gynecology* 139 (1981): 277–80.

4. V. T. Brandeis and S. Bernstein, "Measuring Your Patient's Menstrual Flow," *Contemporary Ob/Gyn*, January 1985, pp. 87–98.

5. M. L. Taymor, S. H. Sturgis, and C. Yahia, "The Etiological Role of Chronic Iron Deficiency in Production of Menorrhagia," *Journal of the American Medical Association* 187 (1964): 323–27.

6. J. McGarry, "Menorrhagia and Intermenstrual Bleeding," *British Journal of Sexual Medicine*, March 1986, pp. 84–85.

7. D. M. Lithgow and W. M. Politzer, "Vitamin A in the Treatment of Menorrhagia," *South African Medical Journal* 51 (1977): 191–93.

8. Editorial, "Vitamin A and Teratogenesis," *Lancet*, February 9, 1985, pp. 319–20.

9. E. Kemmann, S. A. Pasquale, and R. Skaf, "Amenorrhea Associated with Carotenemia," *Journal of the American Medical Association* 249 (1983): 926–29.

10. G. Singh et al., letter, "Can Nifedipine Provoke Menorrhagia?" *Lancet*, October 29, 1983, p. 1022.

11. *Physicians' Desk Reference* (Oradell, N.J.: Medical Economics Company, 1985).

12. D. R. Halbert, "Menstrual Delay and Dysfunctional Uterine Bleeding Associated with Antiprostaglandin Therapy for Dysmenorrhea," *Journal of Reproductive Medicine* 28 (1983): 592–94.

13. O. Ylikorkala and F. Pekonen, "Naproxen Reduces Idiopathic but Not Fibromyoma-Induced Menorrhagia," *Obstetrics and Gynecology* 68 (1986): 10–12.

14. P. B. Pendergrass et al., "The Effect of an H1 Blocker, Chlorpheniramine Maleate, on Total Menstrual Loss," *Gynecologic and Obstetric Investigation* 18 (1984): 238–43.

15. R. S. Ledward, "Low Dose Danazol in Menorrhagia: Four Case Reports," *British Journal of Clinical Practice*, June 1984, pp. 237–38.

16. R. W. Shaw and H. M. Fraser, "Use of a Superactive Luteinizing

Hormone Releasing Hormone (LHRH) Agonist in the Treatment of Menorrhagia," *British Journal of Obstetrics and Gynaecology* 91 (1984): 913–16.

17. L. Nilsson and G. Rybo, "Treatment of Menorrhagia," *American Journal of Obstetrics and Gynecology* 110 (1971): 713–20.

18. R. F. Harrison and S. Campbell, "A Double-Blind Trial of Ethamsylate in the Treatment of Primary and Intrauterine-Device Menorrhagia," *Lancet,* August 7, 1976, pp. 283–85.

19. F. Tudiver, "Dysfunctional Uterine Bleeding and Prior Life Stress," *Journal of Family Practice* 17 (1983): 999–1003; D. D. Youngs and N. Reame, "Psychosomatic Aspects of Menstrual Dysfunction," *Clinical Obstetrics and Gynecology* 26 (1983): 777–84.

20. D. R. Meldrum, "Perimenopausal Menstrual Problems," *Clinical Obstetrics and Gynecology* 26 (1983): 762–68.

21. *Physicians' Desk Reference,* p. 1365.

22. M. H. Goldrath, T. A. Fuller, and S. Segal, "Laser Photovaporization of Endometrium for the Treatment of Menorrhagia," *American Journal of Obstetrics and Gynecology* 140 (1980): 14–19; J. Daniell, R. Tosh, and S. Meisels, "Photodynamic Ablation of the Endometrium with the Nd:YAG Laser Hysteroscopically as a Treatment of Menorrhagia," *Colposcopy and Gynecologic Laser Surgery* 2 (1986): 43–46.

23. Y. C. Choo et al., "Postmenopausal Uterine Bleeding of Nonorganic Cause," *Obstetrics and Gynecology* 66 (1985): 225–28.

24. J. Dewhurst, "Postmenopausal Bleeding from Benign Causes," *Clinical Obstetrics and Gynecology* 26 (1983): 769–76.

CHAPTER 6. *Hyperplasia and Endometrial Cancer*

1. H. S. Page and A. J. Asire, *Cancer Rates and Risks,* NIH Publication No. 85–691, National Cancer Institute, 3rd ed., 1985.

2. M. P. Connor and H. J. Norris, "Which Tumors Are Mostly Benign?" *Contemporary Ob/Gyn,* April 1986, pp. 41–45; J. D. Crissman, et al., "Endometrial Carcinoma in Women 40 Years of Age or Younger," *Obstetrics and Gynecology* 57 (1981): 699; A. Ferenczy and M. M. Gelfand, "Hyperplasia Versus Neoplasia: Two Tracks for the Endometrium?" *Contemporary Ob/Gyn,* August, 1986, pp. 79–94.

3. L. G. Koss et al., "Screening of Asymptomatic Women for Endometrial Cancer," *Obstetrics and Gynecology* 57 (1981): 681–91.

4. S. Shapiro et al., "Risks of Localized and Widespread Endometrial

Cancer in Relation to Recent and Discontinued Use of Conjugated Estrogens," *New England Journal of Medicine* 313 (1985): 969–72.

5. S. M. Lesko et al., "Cigarette Smoking and the Risk of Endometrial Cancer," *New England Journal of Medicine* 313 (1985): 594–600.

6. N. C. Siddle, "How Progestins Prevent Endometrial Cancer," *Revue Française de Gynecologie et d'Obstetrique* 80 (1985): 219–21.

7. D. Gal et al., "Long-term Effect of Megestrol Acetate in the Treatment of Endometrial Hyperplasia," *American Journal of Obstetrics and Gynecology* 146 (1983): 316–22.

8. R. E. Fechner and R. H. Kaufman, "Endometrial Adenocarcinoma in Stein-Leventhal Syndrome," *Cancer* 34 (1974): 444–52; W. A. Eddy, "Endometrial Carcinoma in Stein-Leventhal Syndrome Treated with Hydroxyprogesterone Caproate," *American Journal of Obstetrics and Gynecology* 131 (1978): 581–82; J. V. Bokhman et al., "Can Primary Endometrial Carcinoma Stage I Be Cured Without Surgery and Radiation Therapy?" *Gynecologic Oncology* 20 (1985): 139–55; J. G. Thornton et al., "Primary Treatment of Endometrial Cancer with Progestagen Alone," *Lancet*, July 27, 1985, pp. 207–8.

9. R. J. Kurman, P. F. Kaminski, and H. J. Norris, "The Behavior of Endometrial Hyperplasia: A Long-Term Study of 'Untreated' Hyperplasia in 170 Patients," *Cancer* 56 (1985): 403–12.

10. W. T. Creasman et al., "Estrogen Replacement Therapy in the Patient Treated for Endometrial Cancer," *Obstetrics and Gynecology* 67 (1986): 326–30.

11. E. Saksela, V. Lampinen, and B.-J. Procope, "Malignant Mesenchymal Tumors of the Uterine Corpus," *American Journal of Obstetrics and Gynecology* 120 (1974): 452–60; J. B. Wheelock et al., "Uterine Sarcoma: Analysis of Prognostic Variables in 71 Cases," *American Journal of Obstetrics and Gynecology* 151 (1984): 1016–22; K. V. Kahanpaa et al., "Sarcomas of the Uterus: A Clinicopathologic Study of 119 Patients," *Obstetrics and Gynecology* 67 (1986): 417–24.

12. J. M. Heath, T. H. Bu, and W. F. Brereton, "Hydatidiform Moles," *American Family Physician* 31 (1985): 123–31; K. D. Bagshawe, "Treatment of High-Risk Choriocarcinoma," *Journal of Reproductive Medicine* 29 (1984): 813–20; L. C. Wong, Y. C. Choo, and H. K. Ma, "Use of Oral VP16–213 as Primary Chemotherapeutic Agent in Treatment of Gestational Trophoblastic Disease," *American Journal of Obstetrics and Gynecology* 150 (1984): 924–27.

CHAPTER 7. *Cervical Changes, Including Cancer*

1. S. B. Sadeghi, E. W. Hsieh, and S. W. Gunn, "Prevalence of Cervical Intraepithelial Neoplasia in Sexually Active Teenagers and Young Adults," *American Journal of Obstetrics and Gynecology* 148 (1984): 726–29.

2. R. M. Richart, "Colpomicroscopic Studies of Cervical Intraepithelial Neoplasia," *Cancer* 19 (1966): 395–405.

3. L. G. Koss et al., "Some Histological Aspects of Behavior of Epidermoid Carcinoma in Situ and Related Lesions of the Uterine Cervix," *Cancer* 9 (1963): 1160–1211; L. J. Kinlen and A. I. Spriggs, "Women with Positive Cervical Smears but Without Surgical Intervention," *Lancet,* August 26, 1978, pp. 463–65.

4. C. La Vecchia et al., " 'Pap' Smear and the Risk of Cervical Neoplasia: Quantitative Estimates from a Case-Control Study," *Lancet,* October 6, 1984, pp. 779–82.

5. L. G. Koss, "Dysplasia: A Real Concept or a Misnomer?" *Obstetrics and Gynecology* 51 (1978): 374–79.

6. W. A. McIndoe et al., "The Invasive Potential of Carcinoma in Situ of the Cervix," *Obstetrics and Gynecology* 64 (1984): 451–58.

7. E. Hemmingsson, U. Stendahl, and S. Stenson, "Cryosurgical Treatment of Cervical Intraepithelial Neoplasia with Follow-Up of Five to Eight Years," *American Journal of Obstetrics and Gynecology* 139 (1981): 144–47; V. C. Wright, E. Davies, and M. A. Riopelle, "Laser Surgery for Cervical Intraepithelial Neoplasia: Principles and Results," *American Journal of Obstetrics and Gynecology* 145 (1983): 181–84; H. J. Kwikkel et al., "Laser or Cryotherapy for Cervical Intraepithelial Neoplasia: A Randomized Study to Compare Efficacy and Side Effects," *Gynecologic Oncology* 22 (1985): 23–31.

8. I. E. Lowles, A. Al-Kurdi, and M. J. Hare, "Women's Recollection of Pain During and After Carbon Dioxide Laser Treatment to the Uterine Cervix," *British Journal of Obstetrics and Gynaecology* 90 (1983): 1157–59.

9. R. Richart, "The Patient with an Abnormal Pap Smear—Screening Techniques and Management," *New England Journal of Medicine* 302 (1980): 332–34.

10. Ibid., p. 333.

11. A. D. Claman and N. Lee, "Factors That Relate to Complications of Cone Biopsy," *American Journal of Obstetrics and Gynecology* 120 (1974): 124–28.

12. G. Larsson, "Historical Background and Introduction: The Con-

ization Operation and Its Predecessors," *Acta Obstetrica et Gynecologica Scandinavica* 114 (1983, suppl.): 7–40.

13. G. B. Kristensen, "The Outcome of Pregnancy and Preterm Delivery After Conization of the Cervix," *Archives of Gynecology* 236 (1985): 127.

14. T. Kuoppala and S. Saarikoski, "Pregnancy and Delivery After Cone Biopsy of the Cervix," *Archives of Gynecology* 237 (1986): 149–54; J. M. Jones, P. Sweetnam, and B. M. Hibbard, "The Outcome of Pregnancy After Cone Biopsy of the Cervix: A Case-Control Study," *British Journal of Obstetrics and Gynaecology* 86 (1979): 913–16; T. Weber and E. Obel, "Pregnancy Complications Following Conization of the Uterine Cervix," *Acta Obstetrica et Gynecologica Scandinavica* 58 (1979): 259–63.

15. Editorial comment on "The Outcome of Pregnancy and Preterm Delivery After Conization of the Cervix," *Obstetrical and Gynecological Survey* 41 (1986): 162–63.

16. M. S. Baggish, "A Comparison Between Laser Excisional Conization and Laser Vaporization for the Treatment of Cervical Intraepithelial Neoplasia," *American Journal of Obstetrics and Gynecology* 155 (1986): 39–44.

17. G. Larsson, P. Alm, and H. Grundsell, "Laser Conization Versus Cold-Knife Conization," *Surgery, Gynecology, and Obstetrics* 154 (1982): 59–61.

18. W. T. Creasman et al., "Management of Stage 1A Carcinoma of the Cervix." *American Journal of Obstetrics and Gynecology* 153 (1985): 164–71.

19. G. A. Webb, "The Role of Ovarian Conservation in the Treatment of Carcinoma of the Cervix with Radical Surgery," *American Journal of Obstetrics and Gynecology* 122 (1975): 476–84.

20. N. Kadar and J. H. Nelson, Jr., "Treatment of Urinary Incontinence After Radical Hysterectomy," *Obstetrics and Gynecology* 64 (1984): 400–5; R. J. Scotti et al., "Urodynamic Changes in Urethrovesical Function After Radical Hysterectomy," *Obstetrics and Gynecology* 68 (1986): 111–20.

21. "Less Radical Surgery in Female Cancers Urged," *Medical Post,* October 21, 1986, p. 38; R. Sutherland, "When Treating Gynecological Cancer: 'Preserve the Childbearing Function,' " *Medical Post,* June 3, 1986, p. 32.

22. W. H. Decker and E. Schwartzman, "Sexual Function Following Treatment for Carcinoma of the Cervix," *American Journal of Obstetrics and Gynecology* 83 (1962): 401–5.

23. A. G. Amias, "Sexual Life After Gynaecological Operations—1," *British Medical Journal,* June 14, 1975, pp. 608–9.

24. M. Hoffman, W. S. Roberts, and D. Cavanagh, "Second Pelvic Malignancies Following Radiation Therapy for Cervical Cancer," *Obstetrical and Gynecological Survey* 40 (1985): 611–17.

25. J. H. Ferguson, "Effect of Stilbestrol on Pregnancy Compared to the Effect of a Placebo," *American Journal of Obstetrics and Gynecology* 65 (1953): 592–601.

26. "DES Daughters: The Risks in Their Childbearing Years," *Contemporary Ob/Gyn,* July 1985, pp. 204–28.

27. C. N. Hudson et al., "Preservation of Reproductive Potential in Diethylstilbestrol-Related Vaginal Adenocarcinoma," *American Journal of Obstetrics and Gynecology* 145 (1983): 375–77.

28. J. T. Wharton et al., "Treatment of Clear-Cell Adenocarcinoma in Young Females," *Obstetrics and Gynecology* 45 (1975): 365–68.

29. C. P. Crum et al., "Human Papillomavirus Type 16 and Early Cervical Neoplasia," *New England Journal of Medicine* 310 (1984): 880–83; "Condyloma Virus and Cervical Cancer—How Strong a Link?" *Contemporary Ob/Gyn,* February 1984, pp. 210–24.

30. R. U. Levine et al., "Cervical Papillomavirus Infection and Intraepithelial Neoplasia: A Study of Male Sexual Partners," *Obstetrics and Gynecology* 64 (1984): 16–20; M. J. Campion et al., "Increased Risk of Cervical Neoplasia in Consorts of Men with Penile Condylomata Acuminata," *Lancet,* April 27, 1985, pp. 943–46.

31. J. Robinson, "Cancer of the Cervix: Occupational Risks of Husbands and Wives and Possible Preventive Strategies," in J. A. Jordon, F. Sharp, and A. Singer, eds., *Pre-Clinical Neoplasia of the Cervix* (London: Royal College of Obstetricians and Gynaecologists, 1982), pp. 11–27.

32. J. R. Daling, K. J. Sherman, and N. S. Weiss, "Risk Factors for Condyloma Acuminatum in Women," *Sexually Transmitted Diseases* 13 (1986): 16–18; O. Lechky, "More Mutagens Seen in Smokers' Cervical Fluid," *Medical Post,* May 14, 1985, p. 27.

33. E. Stern et al., "Steroid Contraceptive Use and Cervical Dysplasia: Increased Risk of Progression," *Science* 196 (1977): 1460–62. M. P. Vessey et al., "Neoplasia of the Cervix Uteri and Contraception: A Possible Adverse Effect of the Pill," *Lancet,* October 22, 1983, pp. 930–34.

34. C. La Vecchia et al., "Dietary Vitamin A and the Risk of Invasive Cervical Cancer," *International Journal of Cancer* 34 (1984): 319–22.

35. "Pap Smear Screening in the US, UK, and Canada," *Contemporary Ob/Gyn,* June 1985, pp. 171–93.

36. S. W. Hall and J. M. Monaghan, "Invasive Carcinoma of the Cervix in Younger Women," *Lancet,* September 24, 1983, p. 731.

37. La Vecchia et al., " 'Pap' Smear and the Risk of Cervical Neoplasia."

38. R. Richart, "The Patient with an Abnormal Pap Smear—Screening Techniques and Management," *New England Journal of Medicine* 302 (1980): 332–34; A. Ferenczy, "Screening for Cervical Cancer: a Renewed Plea for Annual Smears," *Contemporary Ob/Gyn,* July 1986, pp. 93–108.

CHAPTER 8. *Saving Your Ovaries*

1. P. G. Stumpf, "Prophylactic Hysterectomy at Oophorectomy in Young Women," *Journal of the American Medical Association* 252 (1984): 1129–30; D. Navot et al., "Artificially Induced Endometrial Cycles and Establishment of Pregnancies in the Absence of Ovaries," *New England Journal of Medicine* 314 (1986): 806–11.

2. B. Ranney and S. Abu-Ghazaleh, "The Future Function and Fortune of Ovarian Tissue Which Is Retained in Vivo During Hysterectomy," *American Journal of Obstetrics and Gynecology* 128 (1977): 626–34.

3. R. H. Grogan, "Reappraisal of Residual Ovaries," *American Journal of Obstetrics and Gynecology* 97 (1967): 124–29.

4. A. P. M. Heintz, N. F. Hacker and L. D. Lagasse, "Epidemiology and Etiology of Ovarian Cancer: A Review," *Obstetrics and Gynecology* 66 (1985): 127–35.

5. Ibid.

6. M. S. Piver, "Alarming Trends in the Familial Ovarian Cancer Registry," *Contemporary Ob/Gyn,* February 1986, 120–29.

7. K. T. K. Chen, J. L. Schooley, and M. S. Flam, "Peritoneal Carcinomatosis After Prophylactic Oophorectomy in Familial Ovarian Cancer Syndrome," *Obstetrics and Gynecology* 66 (1985 suppl.): 93S–94S.

8. B. L. Dennefors et al., "Steroid Production and Responsiveness to Gonadotropin in Isolated Stromal Tissue of Human Postmenopausal Ovaries," *American Journal of Obstetrics and Gynecology* 136 (1980): 997–1002; C. Longcope, R. Hunter, and C. Franz, "Steroid Secretion by the Postmenopausal Ovary," *American Journal of Obstetrics and Gynecology* 138 (1980): 564–68.

9. C.-R. García and W. B. Cutler, "Preservation of the Ovary: A Reevaluation," *Fertility and Sterility* 42 (1984): 510–14.

10. L. Eriksson, O. Kjellgren and B. von Schoultz, "Functional Cyst or Ovarian Cancer: Histopathological Findings During One Year of Surgery," *Gynecologic and Obstetric Investigation* 19 (1985): 155–59.

11. H. Smedley and K. Sikora, "Age as a Prognostic Factor in Epithelial Ovarian Carcinoma," *British Journal of Obstetrics and Gynaecology* 92 (1985): 839–42.

12. L. Kliman, R. M. Rome, and D. W. Fortune, "Low Malignant Potential Tumors of the Ovary: A Study of 76 Cases," *Obstetrics and Gynecology* 68 (1986): 338–44; D. Barnhill et al., "Epithelial Ovarian Carcinoma of Low Malignant Potential," *Obstetrics and Gynecology* 65 (1985): 53–59; M. Tasker and F. A. Langley, "The Outlook for Women with Borderline Epithelial Tumors of the Ovary," *British Journal of Obstetrics and Gynaecology* 92 (1985): 969.

13. H. Tazelaar et al., "Conservative Treatment of Borderline Ovarian Tumors," *Obstetrics and Gynecology* 66 (1985): 417–22.

14. E. W. Munnell, "Is Conservative Therapy Ever Justified in Stage 1 (1A) Cancer of the Ovary?" *American Journal of Obstetrics and Gynecology* 103 (1969): 641–53.

15. J. R. Lurain, "Confronting Nongestational Ovarian Choriocarcinoma," *Contemporary Ob/Gyn*, March 1985, pp. 67–75; W. T. Creasman et al., "Germ Cell Malignancies of the Ovary," *Obstetrics and Gynecology* 53 (1979): 226–30; S. R. Axe, V. R. Klein, and J. D. Woodruff, "Choriocarcinoma of the Ovary," *Obstetrics and Gynecology* 66 (1985): 111–14.

16. J. P. Micha et al., "Malignant Ovarian Germ-Cell Tumors: A Review of Thirty-Six Cases," *American Journal of Obstetrics and Gynecology* 152 (1985):842–46.

CHAPTER 9. *Pelvic Inflammatory Disease*

1. L. Westrom, "Effects of Acute Pelvic Inflammatory Disease on Fertility," *American Journal of Obstetrics and Gynecology* 121 (1975): 707–13.

2. L. G. Keith et al., "On the Causation of Pelvic Inflammatory Disease," *American Journal of Obstetrics and Gynecology* 149 (1984): 215–24.

3. A. M. Kaunitz and D. A. Grimes, "Good News About Contraceptives and PID," *Contemporary Ob/Gyn*, March 1986, pp. 153–57.

4. William C. Scott, "Pelvic Abscess in Association with Intrauterine Contraceptive Device," *American Journal of Obstetrics and Gynecology* 131 (1978): 149–56.

5. D. A. Grimes et al., "Antibiotic Treatment of Pelvic Inflammatory Disease," *Journal of the American Medical Association* 256 (1986): 3223–26; P. B. Mead, "PID: A Critique of Current Therapies," *Contemporary Ob/Gyn*, August 1985, pp. 111–21.

6. Kaunitz and Grimes, "Good News About Contraceptives and PID."

7. Grimes et al., "Antibiotic Treatment of Pelvic Inflammatory Disease."

8. D. V. Landers and R. L. Sweet, "Tubo-ovarian Abscess: Contemporary Approach to Management," *Reviews of Infectious Diseases* 5 (1983): 876–84.

9. W. Roberts and J. L. Dockery, "Operative and Conservative Treatment of Tubo-ovarian Abscess Due to Pelvic Inflammatory Disease," *Southern Medical Journal* 77 (1984): 860–63.

10. M. E. Rivlin and J. A. Hunt, "Ruptured Tubovarian Abscess: Is Hysterectomy Necessary?" *Obstetrics and Gynecology* 50 (1977): 518–22.

11. Weström, "Effects of Acute Pelvic Inflammatory Disease on Fertility."

12. Ibid.

13. J. G. Hallatt, "Tubal Conservation in Ectopic Pregnancy: A Study of 200 Cases," *American Journal of Obstetrics and Gynecology* 154 (1986): 1216–21.

CHAPTER 10. *Pain—Menstrual, Sexual, and Chronic*

1. D. A. Drossman, "Patients with Psychogenic Abdominal Pain: Six Years' Observation in the Medical Setting," *American Journal of Psychiatry* 139 (1982): 1549–57; J. C. Slocumb, "Neurological Factors in Chronic Pelvic Pain: Trigger Points and the Abdominal Pelvic Pain Syndrome," *American Journal of Obstetrics and Gynecology* 149 (1984): 536–43; C. T. Backstrom, H. Boyle, and D. T. Baird, "Persistence of Symptoms of Premenstrual Tension in Hysterectomized Women," *British Journal of Obstetrics and Gynaecology* 88 (1981): 530–36.

2. A. J. Kresch et al., "Laparoscopy in 100 Women With Chronic Pelvic Pain," *Obstetrics and Gynecology* 64 (1984): 672–74; A. J. Kresch, D. B. Seifer, and J. F. Steege, "How to Manage Patients with Chronic Pelvic Pain," *Contemporary Ob/Gyn*, September 1985, pp. 213–19.

3. R. W. Beard et al., "Diagnosis of Pelvic Varicosities in Women

with Chronic Pelvic Pain," *Lancet,* October 27, 1984, pp. 946–49; R. W. Beard, P. W. Reginald, and S. Pearce, "Pelvic Pain in Women," *British Medical Journal* 293 (1986): 1160–62.

4. Slocumb, "Neurological Factors in Chronic Pelvic Pain."

5. Dr. John C. Slocumb, Department of Obstetrics and Gynecology, University of New Mexico School of Medicine, 2211 Lomas Boulevard N.E., Albuquerque, N.M. 87106.

6. L. R. Malinak, "Pelvic Pain—When Is Surgery Indicated?" *Contemporary Ob/Gyn,* August 1985, pp. 43–51.

7. R. B. Lee et al., "Presacral Neurectomy for Chronic Pelvic Pain," *Obstetrics and Gynecology* 68 (1986): 517–21.

8. W. J. Mann and V. G. Stenger, "Uterine Suspension Through the Laparoscope," *Obstetrics and Gynecology* 51 (1978): 563–66; S. F. Gordon, "Laparscopic Uterine Suspension," Abstracts, Xth World Congress of Gynecology and Obstetrics, San Francisco, Calif., October 17–22, 1982.

9. T. Lundeberg, L. Bondesson, and V. Lundstrom, "Relief of Primary Dysmenorrhea by Transcutaneous Electrical Nerve Stimulation," *Acta Obstetrica et Gynecologica Scandinavica* 64 (1985): 491–97.

CHAPTER 11. *Endometriosis*

1. H. Suginami, K. Hamada, and K. Yano, " A Case of Endometriosis of the Lung Treated With Danazol," *Obstetrics and Gynecology* 66 (1985): 68S–71S.

2. J. Halme et al., "Retrograde Menstruation in Healthy Women and in Patients with Endometriosis," *Obstetrics and Gynecology* 64 (1984): 151.

3. A. Addison et al., "Disposition of the Normal-Appearing Ovary During Surgery Intended to Cure Endometriosis Externa," *Journal of Reproductive Medicine* 29 (1984): 281–83.

4. Personal communication from Dr. J. Daniell.

5. J. Daniell, "Laser Laparoscopy for Endometriosis," *Colposcopy and Gynecologic Laser Surgery* 1 (1984): 185–92.

6. J. Daniell, "Operative Laparoscopy for Endometriosis," *Seminars in Reproductive Endocrinology* 3 (1985): 353–59.

7. "Laparoscopic Laser Ablation Useful Even in Severe Endometriosis," *Ob. Gyn. News,* March 1–14, 1986; "The Laser and Endometriosis," *Endometriosis Association Newsletter,* September–October 1985.

8. N. H. Lauersen, K. H. Wilson, and S. Birnbaum, "Danazol: An

Antigonadotropic Agent in the Treatment of Pelvic Endometriosis,'' *American Journal of Obstetrics and Gynecology* 123 (1975): 742–47.

9. P. A. Mercaitis, R. E. Peaper, and P. A. Schwartz, ''Effect of Danazol on Vocal Pitch: A Case Study,'' *Obstetrics and Gynecology* 65 (1985): 131–35.

10. M. Small et al., ''Danazol and Oral Anticoagulants,'' *Scottish Medical Journal* 27 (1982): 331–32.

11. E. Schriock et al., ''Treatment of Endometriosis with a Potent Agonist of Gonadotropin-Releasing Hormone (Nafarelin),'' *Fertility and Sterility* 44 (1985): 583–88.

CHAPTER 12. *Prolapse—Return of the Pessary?*

1. L. Van Dongen, ''The Anatomy of Genital Prolapse,'' *South African Medical Journal* 60 (1981): 357.

2. J. D. Thompson and H. W. Birch, ''Indications for Hysterectomy,'' *Clinical Obstetrics and Gynecology* 24 (1981): 1250.

3. D. T. Y. Liu, ''Narrowed Introitus,'' *British Journal of Sexual Medicine,* August 1986, p. 242.

4. A. G. Amias, ''Sexual Life After Gynaecological Operations—II,'' *British Medical Journal* 1975, 2: 680–81.

5. A. Koppe et al., ''A Vaginal Approach to the Treatment of Genital Prolapse,'' *European Journal of Obstetrics, Gynecology, and Reproductive Biology* 16 (1984): 359–64.

6. Amias, ''Sexual Life After Gynaecological Operations—II.''

7. Koppe et al., ''A Vaginal Approach to the Treatment of Genital Prolapse.''

8. V. Bonney, ''The Principles That Should Underlie All Operations for Prolapse,'' *Journal of Obstetrics and Gynaecology of the British Empire* 41 (1934): 669–93.

9. A. Dickins, ''Uterine Ligaments and the Treatment of Prolapse,'' *Journal of the Royal Society of Medicine* 77 (1984): 353–56.

10. J. S. Crawford, ''Letter: Episiotomy,'' *British Medical Journal* 284 (1982): 594; R. Hodgkinson, ''Letter: Episiotomy,'' *British Medical Journal* 284(1982): 1042.

11. H. Gordon and M. Logue, ''Perineal Muscle Function After Childbirth,'' *Lancet,* July 20, 1985, pp. 123–25.

12. A. H. Kegel, ''Early Genital Relaxation: New Techniques of Di-

agnosis and Nonsurgical Treatment," *Obstetrics and Gynecology* 8 (1956): 545–50.

13. A. K. Ladas, B. Whipple, and J. D. Perry, *The G Spot: And Other Recent Discoveries About Human Sexuality* (New York: Dell Publishing Co., 1983).

14. I. L. C. Fergusson, "Major Common Problems: Genital Prolapse," *British Journal of Hospital Medicine,* July 1981, pp. 69–72.

15. Van Dongen, "The Anatomy of Genital Prolapse."

16. T. A. Rodenberg, "Pessaries and Prolapse," *Journal of the Florida Medical Association* 68 (1981): 895–97.

CHAPTER 13. *A Patient's Bill of Rights*

1. I. M. Rutkow, "Obstetric and Gynecologic Operations in the United States, 1979 to 1984," *Obstetrics and Gynecology* 67 (1986): 755–59.

Index

O4